HOSPITALIZED CHILDREN AND BOOKS:

a guide for librarians, families, and caregivers

Second Edition

by
MARCELLA F. ANDERSON

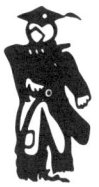

The Scarecrow Press, Inc.
Metuchen, N.J., & London
1992

First edition was published as *Books and Children in Pediatric Settings: A Guide for Caregivers and Librarians.* Copyright 1988 by Marcella F. Anderson. Published under the auspices of Rainbow Babies and Childrens Hospital, through a grant from The Sedgwick Fund, Cleveland, Ohio, 1988.

Illustrator: Ky Wilson
Photographer: Colin Klein

All royalties from this book benefit the library program at Rainbow Babies and Childrens Hospital, Cleveland, OH.

British Library Cataloguing-in-Publication data available

Library of Congress Cataloging-in-Publication Data

Anderson, Marcella F., 1933-
    Hospitalized children and books : a guide for librarians, families, and caregivers / by Marcella F. Anderson. -- 2nd ed.
        p.   cm.
    Rev. ed. of: Books and children in pediatric settings. 1st ed. 1988.
    Includes bibliographical references and indexes.
    ISBN 0-8108-2519-8
    1. Hospital libraries--Activity programs.   2. Hospital patients--Books and reading.   3. Sick children--Books and reading.   4. Children--Hospital care.
    I. Anderson, Marcella F.,   1933-   Books and children in pediatric settings.   II . Title.
    Z675.H7A538   1992
    027.6'62083--dc20   91-41698

Printed on acid-free paper

This book is dedicated to the staff, trustees, and volunteers at Rainbow Babies and Childrens Hospital, especially to the child life specialists for their support of the library program and to Polly B. White, trustee and longtime library committee chairman.

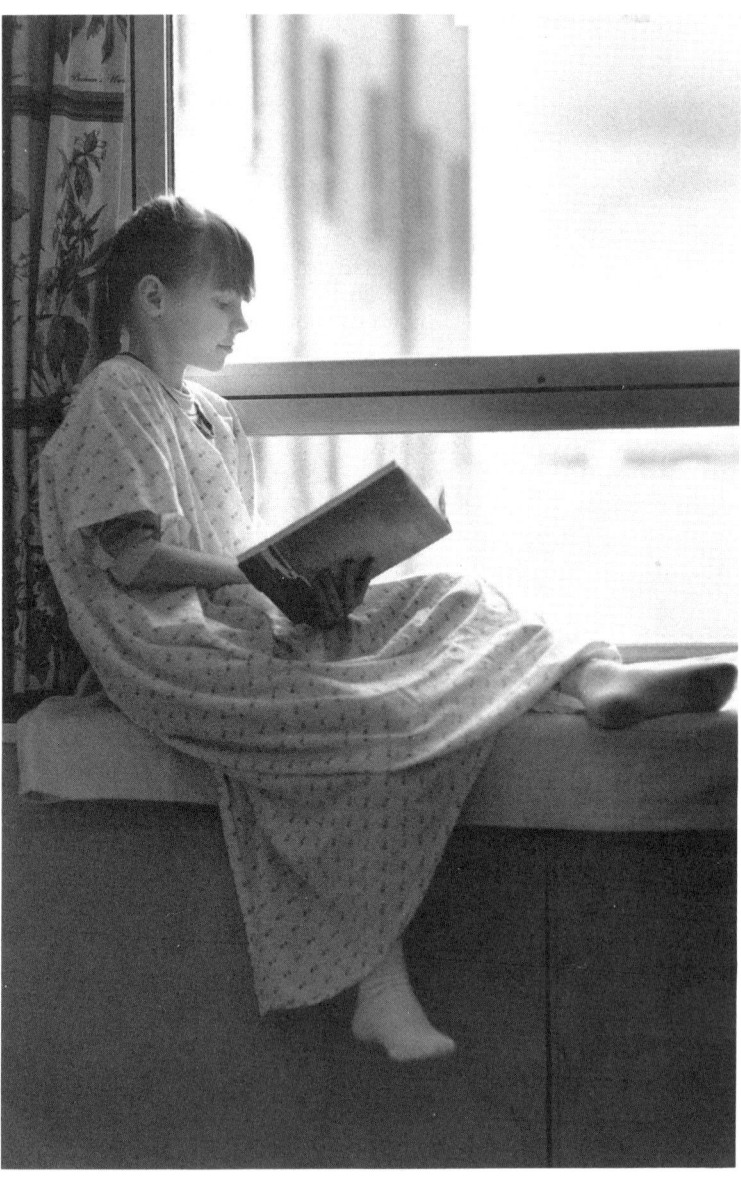

Contents

Contents

Acknowledgments

No book like this one is written alone. I wish to extend my thanks to all who have contributed to its final form.

I am grateful to the following certified child life specialists, who offered valuable content suggestions to individual chapters. My thanks go to: C. Caryn Alfred, B.A.; Mary E. Barkey, M.A.; Mary K. Bowers, B.A.; Tammy Bialik-Bukovec, B.S.; Lisa C. Ginley, B.A.; Alyson L. Grossman, B.S.; Eileen M. Haller, B.S.; Sally A. Niklas, M.A.; Elizabeth A. Ray, M.A.; and Bonnie J. Spitznagel, B.S.

I am particularly indebted to readers of the entire manuscript: Ellen Carr, M.S.; Lauren G. McAliley, M.S.N., R.N.C.; Barbara L. Messner, M.L.S.; and Coleen Olson, M.S. Each contributed insights from the unique perspective of her professional expertise.

Fellow librarians in pediatric settings were generous in taking time from busy schedules to respond to my requests for information. I am grateful to: Lois Alexander, Children's Hospital of Alabama, Birmingham, AL; Kathy Bachmann, Children's Hospital Medical Center of Akron, Akron, OH; Ruby Dillon, Cook-Fort Worth Children's Medical Center, Fort Worth, TX; Barbara Fields, Children's Hospital Oakland, Oakland, CA; Suzanne Flint, The Lucille Salter Packard Children's Hospital at Stanford, Stanford, CA; Karen Nakamura, Carson Regional Library/Harbor UCLA Medical Center, Carson, CA; Taryn Oestreich, Children's Hospital and Medical Center, Seattle, WA; Kathleen Perez, Florida Diagnostic and Learning Resource System, Tampa, FL; Kathy Werner, Phoenix Children's Hospital, Phoenix, AZ; Jerriane Wilson, Johns Hopkins Hospital Children's Center, Baltimore, MD.

To librarians Lynn Dunnagan, Riley Children's Hospital, Indianapolis, IN, and Lyn Ingersoll, Children's National Medical Center, Washington, DC, go special thanks for critiquing specific chapters.

Especially, I wish to acknowledge Elizabeth Crocker, M.Ed., immediate past president of the Association for the Care of Children's Health (ACCH), for her perceptions of the book's initial outline and

ix

Barbara Steele, M.S.W., National Center for Family-Centered Care, for her invaluable information from the patient/family librarian network.

Further thanks go to Helen C. Henry, for her contributions to multicultural titles listed and for her careful reading of the Introduction and Conclusion. I am indebted to all of the following: Paule N. Botkin, M.A., who contributed book reviews and helpful annotations; Mary Jane Neilson, B.A., former library volunteer who contributed experiential insights to a specific chapter; Sylvia Snyder, M.S., who made helpful suggestions to the hospital school segment; and Dalia M. Zemaityte, R.N., M.S.N., who reviewed a specific chapter.

Members of the Rainbow Children's Council, Kathy Stellato and Jennifer Sullivan contributed personal experiences from their book cart service on the patient floors. I am indebted to them and to all Council members for their support of the library.

My thanks go to Lissa Weller, owner of Jabberwocky Children's Bookstore for her helpful interest in this project and to Mercier Robinson, M.L.S. for her assistance in developing programs for Preschool Story Hours.

For the helpful glossary of medical terms, I am grateful to Richard C. Distad, M.D.

My sincere appreciation goes to Donald R. Saunders and T. Ryburn Taylor for patiently guiding me through the intricacies of the personal computer.

My colleagues with the Cuyahoga County Public Library System, Cleveland, OH, have contributed longtime support to the hospital's library program. In particular, I wish to thank Franziska van der Schalie, M.L.S., children's librarian, Orange Branch, for her information and enthusiasm for this project. My appreciation goes also to Jackie Albers, M.L.S., children's librarian, Beachwood Branch and member of the Committee for Library Service to Children with Special Needs, American Library Association (ALA). Her encouragement helped me to embark on the writing of this second edition.

Special acknowledgment is given to Bob Fuller, graphic designer, who volunteered his expertise to the layout of this book.

To Robin Van Kannel of Master Printing Company, thank you for your skills, accurate corrections, and steady hand.

I am deeply grateful to my library volunteers: Armine G. Cuber, whose reading of the second proof provided a final clarification of the text, and to Marie W. Fasig, whose precise work assisted in preparing the index. Thank you for your loyalty and dedication to the library program. Appreciation is expressed also to library intern Janine F. Obee, who assisted in all aspects of the program and added a particular joy to our work during the preparation of this book.

I am further grateful to families who permitted photographs of their children to be included in the text.

Once again, I owe a special appreciation to my daughter, Marcella A. Distad, M.L.S. and to longtime friend, Gretchen S. Larson, M.L.S. As editors, they have spent countless hours in an unrelenting search for accuracy.

Finally, my deepest thanks go to my family — my children, their spouses, and grandchildren for their understanding and patience during the past fourteen months. Especially, I wish to thank my husband, Glenn, for planning leisure respites from work on this book and for offering thoughtful encouragement.

Preface

This revised, updated, second edition of *Hospitalized Children and Books — A Guide for Librarians, Families, and Caregivers* was written to fill a growing need for information about the operation, programming, and goals of a library in a pediatric setting.

Further, this edition was written to provide guidelines for serving an increasingly large preschool-age hospital census and to address the needs of a growing population of chronically ill children. The number of children who are technologically dependent has also increased notably. Their needs must be met by adaptations both in library services and programming.

To address these developments, this edition contains five additional chapters. Titles in children's books and available program resources have also been updated.

Introduction:

The Goals and Values of a Patient/ Family Library in a Pediatric Setting

One of the founders of the Child Life profession, Emma Plank, stressed her belief that the "growing child cannot afford to interrupt the cycle of his living and growth" while in the hospital. "The child's normal way of living...has to be skillfully fitted into a day filled with diagnostic and treatment procedures. The task is complicated by the threat of the illness itself, of operations, and the possible nearness of death."[1]

In a pediatric setting, a library program exists so that "the rhythm of life and growth go on...."[2] The components of a library program are:

> Story hours appropriate for specific age groups, using books, flannel board stories, puppetry, filmstrips, music, and creative projects
> Read-aloud times by the librarian, other staff members, and, especially, by volunteers, who are guided by the librarian
> Book cart services to the patient care areas
> Bibliotherapy with identified patients
> Poetry writing time
> A Family Health Resource Center
> Community outreach

Although short-term patients benefit from a library program, the long-term and frequently hospitalized patient should be a major focus of concern. Medical advances have created the technologically dependent child; the child living with chronic illness; the emerging survivor. For these children and young adults and for all hospitalized young patients, a library program that nurtures the child with enriching materials as he or she moves through developmental stages while hospitalized, supports the "fullest possible development and expression of individual potential."[3]

In addition to supporting that potential, the library program — with other pediatric therapies — helps to normalize the hospital experience. In addition, a library program offers therapeutic interventions and insights through individual reading, storytelling, and read-aloud times. It provides also a chance to express emotions and to enhance self-esteem through poetry writing. Finally, the program provides a catalyst to enhance that quality which supports the process of effective treatment and healing.

The guidelines presented in the following chapters represent the practices of a thriving library program at a major children's medical center. The author's observations are the culmination of nearly fifteen years of experience and ongoing education. The contents of this book are presented in consultation with other librarians in other pediatric settings. My thanks for their invaluable input appear in the Acknowledgments.

All names have been changed to protect a child's identity. "Librarian" is used synonymously with "person-in-charge," who may be an individual from another area of expertise. Wherever possible, "he" and "she" are alternated to avoid awkwardness.

All pediatric settings have their own characteristics. Adaptation of this book's material to suit the needs of individual environments and patient populations will result in measurable success.

You are about to enter the world of hospitalized children who are listening to stories, writing poetry, and reading books or magazines. I hope you will find this guide helpful.

Marcella F. Anderson, B.A.
Patient/Family Librarian
Rainbow Babies and Childrens Hospital
The Children's Hospital of
University Hospitals of Cleveland
Cleveland, Ohio

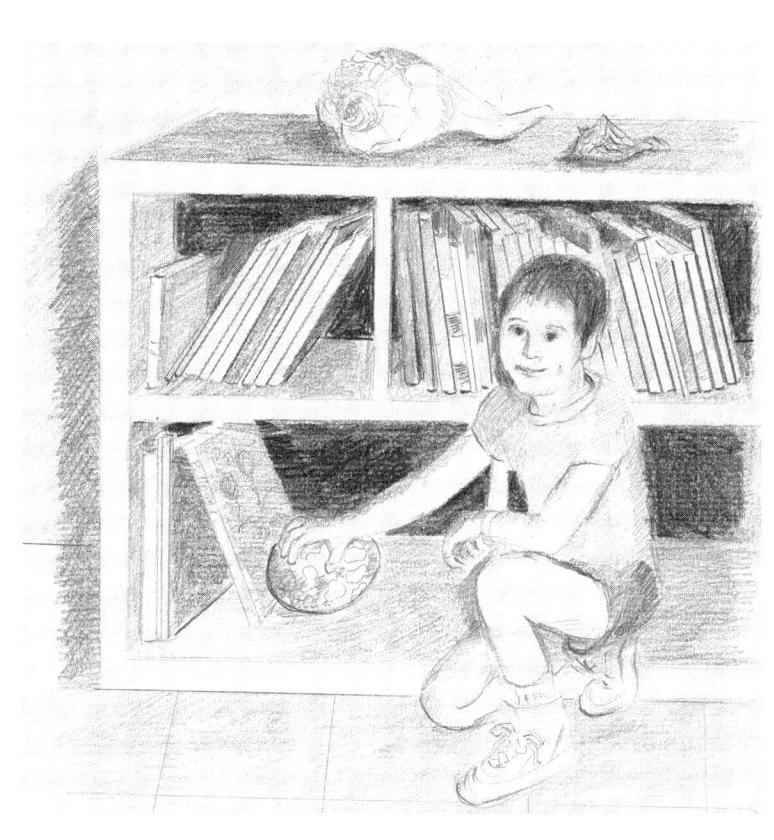

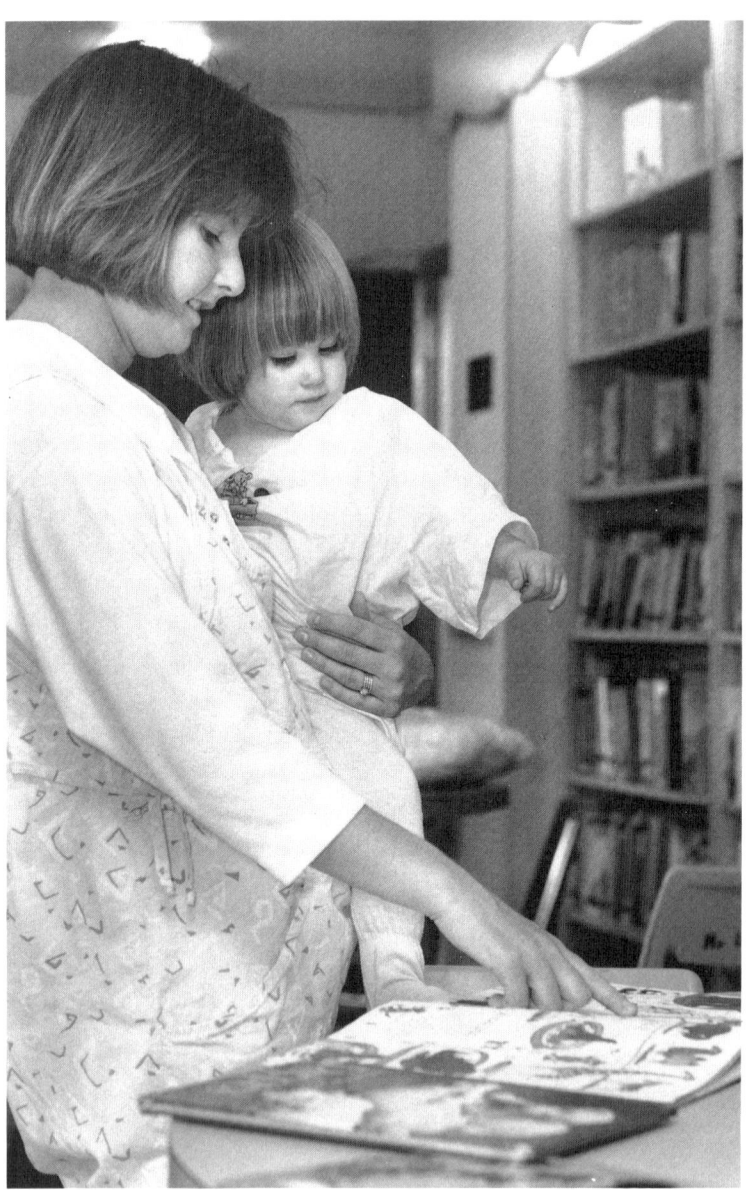

Chapter 1.

ESTABLISHING A LIBRARY PRESENCE IN A CHILDREN'S HOSPITAL

SUPPORT FOR THE CONCEPT

To begin a patient/family library program in a pediatric setting, ascertain early major sources of support. Prepare a carefully conceived and clearly written five-to-ten-year plan with goals and implementations for each year. Explain how a library program will directly benefit the hospital's patients. Be clear in stating the program's specific purposes. Present the plan to a few of the following administrative persons: the hospital administrative medical director; director of pediatric nursing; child life, recreation or play therapy director; director of volunteers; director of public relations and development; head teacher in the school program; president of the hospital trustees, auxillary, and any others who might support your proposal for establishing a library program.

Refer to this book and others as guidelines for establishing a library program. Emphasize that, in addition to books for recreational reading and for information, the library collection will offer sound filmstrips, videos, cassettes, reference books, and books for children with sensory deprivations. Stress also that at least half of the collection will comprise used books donated to the library.

Elicit the interest of the public library. In return, the public library may offer support services and materials. It is especially important to involve early a professional children's librarian and a medical librarian. Their expertise will be invaluable and will add a professional dimension to the library program concept.

Clearly, a hospital is a large, bureaucratic institution. Proposals get shuffled about and sometimes tabled; decision making can be slow; follow-up phone calls are always necessary. Friendly persistence on your part will prove your commitment to the idea.

FUNDING

Financial support for the library program and book collection can come from various sources. Take a comprehensive and visionary approach to fund-raising. Various sources of funding have been used in many pediatric settings. Listed below are a few examples of money sources:

Single or family benefactors
Community service groups, especially Junior Leagues
    and sororities
Honor and memorial gifts
Hospital non-revenue operating budget
Library fundraisers, such as poetry anthologies written
    by patients
Child life, volunteer department, or nursing budgets
Heinz Baby Food labels program
Hospital board or auxillary monies
Children's Miracle Telethon proceeds
Individual community-sponsored fundraisers
Foundation grants — family and community

A few other money sources are:

Library Services Construction Act (L.S.C.A.) grants
"Federal Maternal and Child Health Bureau" grant
Parent groups
State departments of health and education
National Health Foundation
Health and Education Pediatric Department;
    Pediatric Residency Program; United Doctors' Association;
    Nurses Alumnae Association; Committee of Interns and
    Residents
Endowed memorial funds
Corporate grants
State Coalition for the Education of Handicapped Children

FINDING THE SPACE — AND KEEPING IT!

Dedicated library space is essential in order to house the collection, provide a base of operation, and to establish a physical presence in the hospital. Space can be found in a variety of areas. A specifically identified library space is the most desirable. If this is not possible, shared space, such as space shared with a health science library, is a workable option. Be alert to the possibility that space for a library can be designed into future construction.

Finding the space can be less difficult than keeping it. In a hospital-wide space crunch, the library may be sacrificed early. Several stategies may prevent this from happening:

1. Stay close to your source of advocacy within the administration. This practice minimizes surprise decisions that may be sprung on you due to a lack of communication, administrative failure to consider repercussions, or a conscious desire to create a sense of "fait accompli." Supporters must be informed of plans that could jeopardize the library program.

2. Although it may seem to be a contradiction in terms, sharing the space is one way to protect it. Open the library to any and all departments that may need the space for meetings, conferences with families, receptions, and training programs. A written schedule in a central location minimizes conflicts in room use and helps the

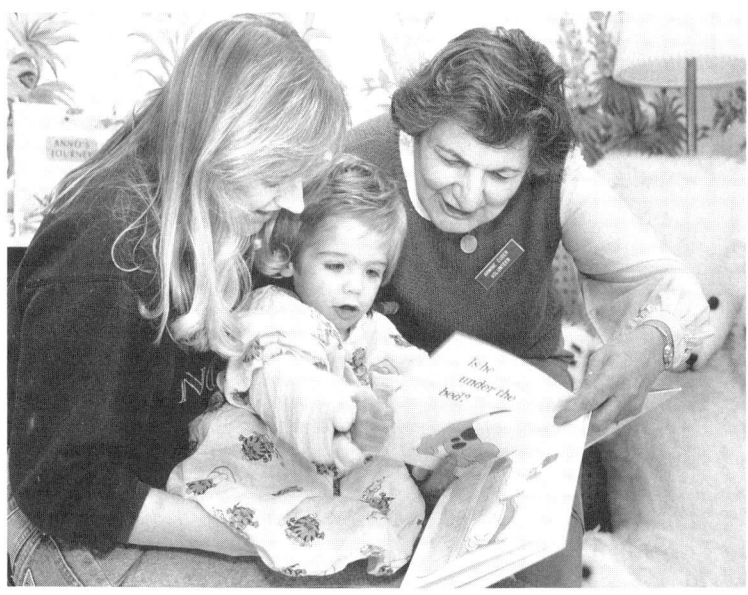

The picture book corner is a favorite area in the library.

librarian plan her schedule. Require that formally scheduled meetings that impinge on your presence be cleared with you. On days with regularly scheduled library programs, such as story hours, the space should not be compromised.

3. Insure that the room stays busy. Child life specialists, volunteers, and teachers are enthusiastic users of the library and its programming. Acquainting the medical, nursing, social work, and dietary staffs with the Family Resource Collection (see Chapter 12) will foster their use of library programming and services.

4. Be creative with new ideas for improving and expanding library services, making the program increasingly significant in meeting the needs of patients, families, and staff.

5. Continue to generate ways in which the library program creates connections for the hospital within the general community. A few examples are: information displays at conferences and at hospital-sponsored events for the community; encouragement of local school projects to collect books for the library collection; willingness to present story hours in community preschools and day care centers.

ORGANIZING THE LIBRARY SPACE

Whatever space has been found as a base of operation for the library program, the processing and shelving of materials plus circulation and access to them should be organized in an uncomplicated manner. (See Chapter 15.)

Materials can be organized according to the Dewey Decimal or Library of Congress Classification. Especially for smaller collections, an informal color coding system works best in many hospitals. A prominently displayed explanatory chart guides the library user in the search for materials. At Children's National Medical Center, Washington, DC, books are color coded based on the numbers in the Dewey Decimal System.

If the library is only staffed part-time but the collection is accessible full-time, choosing books can be simplified by housing popular reading categories on specifically labeled shelves, e.g., mysteries, horses/dogs/cats, early readers, and other interests.

Each book should carry an identifying library bookplate. Honor and memorial books carry commemorative labels as well. At Riley Children's Hospital, IN, memorial bookplates are not used. "Honor" bookplates cover all categories of contribution. Persons interested in making donations are encouraged to contact the librarian to ascertain specific needs.

Encourage a library open door policy as much as security and reason allow. In most hospital settings, circulation and access are available through the librarian, volunteers on the patient floors, and staff members. Book cart service and an open shelf honor system are other means of book access and circulation. At the end of Story Hours, many patients have increased interest in borrowing books.

Some hospitals request that books be signed out. At Children's Hospital Oakland, CA, books are signed out by the date and child's name and floor, not by room number, a constantly changing situation. After three months of no return, the book card is tossed out. To aid program volunteers, books are charged out according to title, instead of author.

Most frequently in pediatric settings, borrowers are not required to sign out books. Instead, they are requested to return books to the book return box on each floor or to the library before leaving the hospital. Because book tracking is not emphasized, book losses do, unfortunately, occur. Reminder bookmarks and posters help to keep losses to a manageable minimum. The Family Resource Collection requires different access procedures, to be explained in Chapter 12.

CREATING AN INVITING ENVIRONMENT

Whatever the space constraints, an important aspect of the library area is its appeal. The young patient is energized by a bright setting and enticing books on display.

For the hospitalized child there are other considerations as well. In contrast to the many anxieties and interruptions on the patient floors, the library is a place where a child can concentrate in a quiet environment, a "safe" place where medical procedures are not permitted.

Guidelines for room design are much the same as for the children's room in public libraries. Ideally, a hospital library should have a window to provide reference to the day's passing; two doors, one wide enough to admit a patient in a bed; child-size chairs plus several adult-size chairs. To accommodate wheelchair patients who may come in alone, unusually high or low shelves should be avoided.

A rationale for the decor created for the hospitalized child is to keep him in touch with the world outside the hospital walls. The young patient needs to be reminded continually that the hospital environment is only part of the world, not the real world from which he comes. Outside, children are swimming, bicycling and going to school — and someday he will again, too. Outside, family and friends are waiting for the child's return.

The natural world is waiting too, though changing. Tadpoles are growing into frogs, green tomatoes are turning red, leaves are falling, snow is in the clouds.

Keeping the patient in contact with the ongoing world enables him to progress cognitively and helps him to think about his place in the world outside the hospital environment. With this in mind, normal activities of childhood, special events, holidays, and seasonal changes should be highlighted in hospital library decor.

SUGGESTED ENHANCERS FOR THE ENVIRONMENT

1. Ask a creative friend or scout troop to do a craft project for the shelves (An eleven-year-old made plaster casts of Beatrix Potter characters; a Sunday-school class made snowmen from white socks for our library).

2. Hang a bulletin board for the patients' artwork and photos. Important notices can be posted as well.

3. Create nature displays: pine cones, shells, feathers — anything a child can pick up and examine. (One spring, a robin's nest was on display. After an inner city child heard that the robin used mud and grass to make her nest, she shouted, "A BIRD made that!").

4. Bring in flowers, and make paper stand-up displays of a farm or house.

5. Purchase a few appropriate posters to brighten the walls. (See Resources)

6. Leave space for one or two fiction or nonfiction books to stand up on display. Signs that say "Display Books May Be Borrowed" encourage circulation.

7. Avoid displaying items of personal or monetary value.

8. In all displays, consider color, harmony, and balance to offset the harsh implements of technology that surround the child and his family.

Chapter 2.

BUILDING THE COLLECTION FOR
THE HOSPITALIZED CHILD

"...Only the rarest kind of best in anything can be good enough for the young."[1] This often-quoted and timeless concept can be the guide to building a core collection of books for hospitalized young readers — especially the chronically ill child who may spend many months of every year hospitalized.

FILLING THE SHELVES

When starting a collection, the librarian should purchase multiple copies of perennial favorites, such as *Peter's Chair* (Keats) and *The Very Busy Spider* (Carle). This is particularly true when working from a "start up" fund where future monies for replacement and expansion are uncertain.

Books that do not circulate in the hospital environment do not deserve a place on the shelves. Hospital libraries have limited space that can be better used for holding multiple copies of favorite books and for shelf displays to pique the child's interest.

Hospital libraries must also have shelf space for foreign language books such as *Curious George Rides a Bike* (Rey) in German. The public library can be especially helpful in providing foreign language books in less commonly spoken languages.

Today, multicultural literature is important in acquainting young readers with various cultural diversities. Some book examples are *In the Year of the Boar and Jackie Robinson* (Lord) and *Arroz Con Leche — Popular Songs and Rhymes from Latin America* (Delacre).

At Cook-Fort Worth Children's Medical Center, Spanish speaking volunteers make book tapes for Hispanic patients to listen to while following along in picture books and easy readers in English.

Special materials for the child with a sensory impairment are recommended also. Books on tape and Braille books are important in the collection. Picture books with illustrated signing are useful in reading aloud to the child with a hearing impairment. (See Resources.)

MAKING BASIC TITLE CHOICES

Keep to high standards. Young readers do not need books "which are condescending, which trivialize their concerns and efforts, and which present easy answers to complex problems...." Instead, they need reality oriented materials to support "their efforts to create meaning in the world."[2]

Children in all circumstances feel their vulnerability, their smallness, and lack of power. Through identifying with book characters, children can experience self-determination, independence, and success. This is especially important for the child who is hospitalized or who is chronically ill. "If we leave [the children] alone to identify with characters...we are allowing the books to work the magic of identification and spread the balm of good therapy on their bruises."[3]

In addition to making book choices with these concepts in mind, it is important to choose book titles appropriate to a child's developmental level. It is also important to choose appropriate materials that address a child's concerns during hospitalization.

The following information may serve as a guideline. It is based on a number of studies combined with the author's personal experience. (See Resources)

INFANTS — 6 months to 18 months

The infant should have an early exposure to books. Reading to a very young child strengthens the bond between child and parent and helps to promote in the young listener a sense of security and trust.

Recommended titles — warmth, sound and rhythm of language, fun with books

Good Night, Moon (Brown, M.W.)
The Little Chick (McCue)
Little Bunny Follows His Nose (Howard)

Moo, Moo, Peekaboo! (Dyer)
Poems to Read to the Very Young (Frank)
Clap Hands (Oxenbury)
All Fall Down (Oxenbury)
The Orchard Book of Nursery Rhymes (Sutherland)
Baby Mother Goose (Fujikawa, il.)
All Through the Night (Boulton)

THE TODDLER — 18 months to 3 years

This age child has strong attachment to parents. During hospitalization, she fears separation and strangers.

Recommended titles — assurance of family love, home, and reunion

Runaway Bunny (Brown, M.W.)
Where's Spot? (Hill)
Say Goodnight (Oxenbury)
Me and My Mom (Slier)
Dad's Back (Ormerod)
How Many Kisses Good Night (Monrad)
Whose Mouse Are You? (Kraus)
Runaway Rabbit (Maris)

The toddler is beginning to gain some autonomy. In the hospital, she loses control over daily routines, activities, and mobility, and may fear she will not regain them.

Recommended titles — support for acquired skills

How Do I Put It On? (Watanabe)
Max's Breakfast (Wells)
The Very Hungry Caterpillar (Carle)
Pat the Bunny (Kunhardt)
Ten, Nine, Eight (Bang)
Tom and Pippo Read a Story plus others in series (Oxenbury)

THE PRESCHOOLER — 3 to 5 years

This age child is beginning to make friendships. In the hospital, he is concerned about relationships that he can trust. He needs books that affirm his having moved away from ego-centeredness to trusting himself and other people, especially in new situations.

Recommended titles — reassurance and trust relationships

Ira Sleeps Over (Waber)
Not So Fast, Songololo (Daly)
Alfie Gets In First and
An Evening At Alfie's (Hughes)
Annabelle Swift, Kindergartner (Schwartz)
Aren't You Coming Too? (Rice)
Just Like Daddy (Asch)

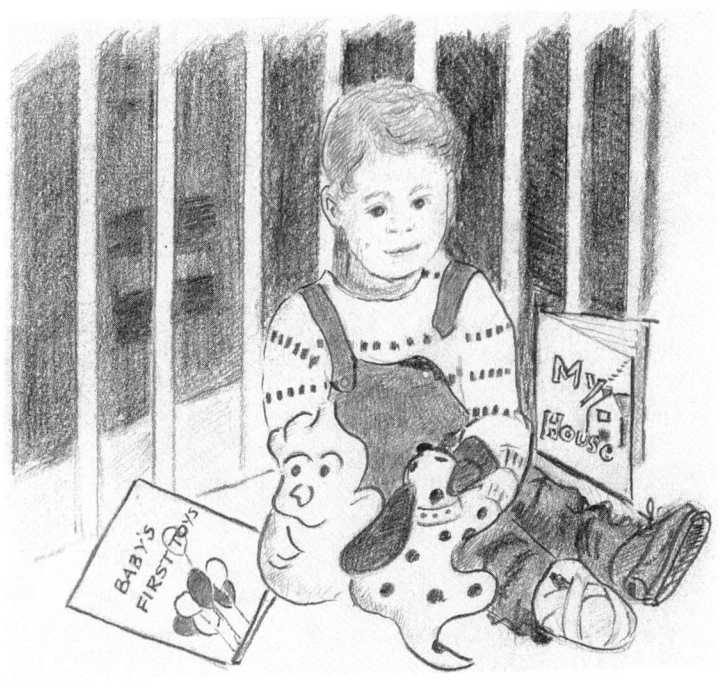

The preschooler still needs reassurance of family and home.
In the hospital, he fears abandonment.

Recommended titles — assurance of family love and
return home

Harry, the Dirty Dog (Zion)
Make Way for Ducklings (McCloskey)
Rosie's Walk (Hutchins)
Ask Mr. Bear (Flack)

We're Going on a Bear Hunt (Rosen)
Big World, Small World (Titherington)
Angel Child, Dragon Child (Surat)
Amifika (Clifton)

Like the toddler, the preschooler has begun acquiring certain skills. He needs reassurance that he will not lose them while in the hospital.

Recommended titles — reaffirmation of skills

Whistle for Willie (Keats)
Swimmy (Lionni)
Anna's Rain (Burstein)
Winter Harvest (Aragon)
Stina (Anderson)
How Many Are in this Old Car? (Hawkins)
Benny Bakes a Cake (Rice)
Anna in Charge (Tsutsui)

The preschooler is curious about the world. It is important that the hospitalized preschooler continue to learn about work and play and the seasons of the year.

Recommended titles — the world outside the hospital

The Listening Walk (Showers)
A Summer Day (Florian)
When Autumn Comes (Maass)
My Spring Robin (Rockwell)
The Snowy Day (Keats)
Bear Child's Book of Special Days (Rockwell)
Farm Morning (McPhail)
The Biggest Truck (Lyon)
Freight Train (Crews)
Out and About (Hughes) — poetry
A Country Far Away (Gray)

In addition, the preschooler is developing his imagination. The hospitalized preschooler needs to escape into fantasy and uses his imagination to help cope with his hospital experience.

Recommended titles — encouragement of developing
imagination

Pretend You're a Cat (Marzollo)
It's Just Me, Emily (Hines)
If I Had a Pig (Inkpen)
Four Brave Sailors (Ginsburg)
Mooncake (Asch)
The Pirates of Bedford Street (Isadora)

THE SCHOOL AGE CHILD — 6 to 12 years

This age child fits also into the pre-adolescent group. The wide
age range and reading levels in this category are to provide flexibility
in meeting the skills and reading interests of the chronically ill child.
The school age child wants information. In the hospital, her general
curiosity should be encouraged.

Recommended titles — informational books

Nicky the Nature Detective (Svedberg)
The Magic School Bus:Inside the Human Body (Cole)

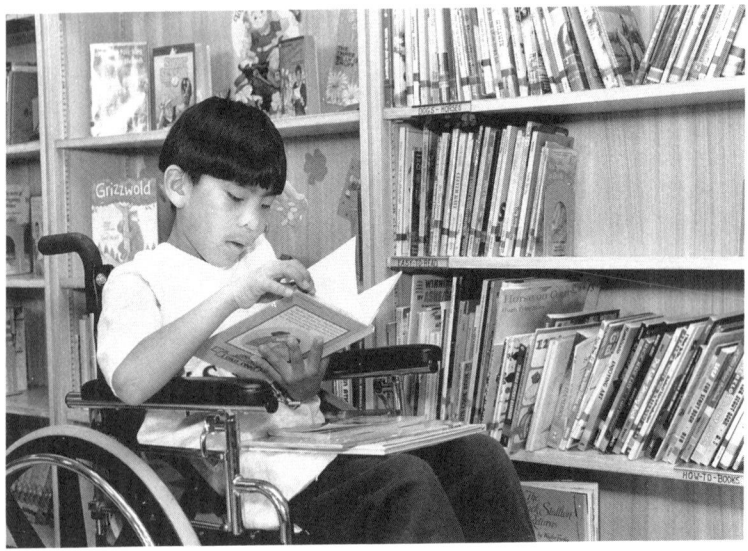

The library is a quiet place to browse through books.

After the Dinosaurs (Shooter)
Exploring the Titanic (Ballard)
Whales (Berger)
Sharks (Berger)
Stars and Planets (Lampton)
The City Kid's Field Guide (Herberman)
Books for World Explorers (National Geographic Society)

In addition, this age child is learning to make choices and to develop a personal set of values. The hospitalized school age child needs access to biographies and to realistic fiction with easily identifiable characters, who are also making choices. "At the very least, realistic fiction offers some interesting views of the often puzzling and disturbing landscape of adolescence. At best it gives readers a chance to explore the terrain and come up with answers of their own." [4]

Recommended titles — testing of values and ideas

Song of the Trees (Taylor)
On My Honor (Bauer)
Ragtime Tumpie (Schroeder)
Lincoln: A Photobiography (Freedman)
The True Confessions of Charlotte Doyle (Avi)

Peer acceptance is very important to the school age child. Loss of peer support is an important concern of the hospitalized child, especially of the long-term patient. Reading a popular author or the latest title in a series enables the hospitalized child to share a common interest with friends both inside and outside the hospital.

Recommended titles — sharing reading with peers

Encyclopedia Brown, Boy Detective plus others in series (Sobol)
Anastasia Krupnik plus others in series (Lowry)
Tales of a Fourth Grade Nothing plus other J/YA series titles (Blume)
The Baby-Sitters Club: Kristy's Great Idea plus others in series (Martin, A.)
A Blossom Promise plus other series titles (Byars)
Bingo Brown and the Language of Love plus other series titles (Byars)
Our Sixth Grade Sugar Babies (Bunting)
Nothing's Fair in Fifth Grade (DeClements)

The People Could Fly (Hamilton)
Baseball in April (Soto)
Making the Team (Hughes, D.) Angel Park All Stars Series

This age child seeks independence and personal achievement. The hospitalized child's opportunities for doing so are limited. Of special importance to this child are survival stories, heroic legends, and myths. These books provide the opportunity for the reader to live the adventure vicariously and to experience through character identification the satisfaction of having survived — and perhaps of having made a difference. Like fairy tales, these books advise the reader: "Take your courage in hand and go out to meet the world head on."[5] The reader learns also that "all survivors bring with them on their return a new strength and certainty" and "that people can find in themselves the courage to go on — not to surrender to despair."[6]

Recommended titles — heroism and survival

Number the Stars (Lowry)
Snow Treasure (McSwigan)
St. George and the Dragon (Hodges)
The Sign of the Beaver (Speare)
Island of the Blue Dolphins (O'Dell)
Call It Courage (Sperry)
Maniac Magee (Spinelli)
Homecoming (Voigt)
Where the Red Fern Grows (Rawls)
My Side of the Mountain and
On the Far Side of the Mountain (George)
The Neverending Story (Ende)
The Road From Home (Kherdian)

PAIN AND STRESS REDUCTION

Humor:

Meeting children's needs through books does not always have to be approached from a serious direction. Humor is often the stuff of life, especially in a pediatric hospital. Studies show that humor helps to reduce stress and to release endorphins, the body's natural pain blockers that lower pain levels and contribute to a sense of well being. Also, humor helps patients to relax by the diversion it offers.[7] The librarian notes this especially in Story Hour. Young patients can be jolted out of sadness and anxiety.

Nearly all children love to laugh and do so without self-consciousness. "Children and humor naturally go together at each stage of their development."[8] The long-term hospitalized preschooler may lack the everyday experiences needed to recognize comedy in ordinary situations, but the short-term hospitalized preschooler will laughingly recognize the ridiculous and nonsensical. The school age child hospitalized for any length of time has a sense of humor waiting to be tickled. No one sees the humorous incongruities in a hospital setting as easily as the school age "hospital child" who has seen it all.

Recommended titles — humor and silliness

The Stupids Step Out (Allard)
Swamp Monsters (Christian)
I Took My Frog to the Library (Kimmel)
Ramona the Pest plus other series titles (Cleary)
Henry and Mudge plus others in series (Rylant)
The Mouse Rap (Myers)
Amelia Bedelia plus others in series (Parish)
Cloudy with a Chance of Meatballs (Barrett)
Miss Nelson is Missing (Allard)
Chicka Chicka Boom Boom (Martin, B. and Archambault)
The Relatives Came (Rylant)
Come a Tide (Lyon)
The Random House Book of Humor for Children (Pollock, ed.)
If This Is Love, I'll Take Spaghetti (Conford)
The B.F.G. (Dahl)
Get Well Clown-Arounds (Cole)
Be a Perfect Person in Just Three Days (Manes)

In addition to humorous books, a collection should be well stocked with joke and riddle books, both of which offer personal relaxation and opportunities for interaction with families, staff, and fellow patients.

Quiet Books:

Quiet books written in a prose poetry style and often beautifully illustrated can help to reduce stress and pain. Certain books offer characters who are themselves reassuring and supportive. These books should also find a place in the collection.

Recommended titles — serenity, reassurance, and beauty

Sarah, Plain and Tall (MacLachlan)
Sailing with the Wind (Locker)
My Prairie Year (Harvey)
Time of Wonder (McCloskey)
Heartland (Siebert)
Stopping By Woods on a Snowy Evening (Frost) — poetry
Bird Watch (Yolen) — poetry
Appalachia: the Voices of Sleeping Birds (Rylant)
Johnny Appleseed (Lindbergh)

Of all prose poetry books, *Owl Moon* (Yolen) is a special gift to a pediatric hospital library. Besides showing a warm relationship between parent and child as well as the natural world on a snowy, moonlight night, the text and illustrations combine at the end to create an almost mystical quality.

A child nearing the end of her short life went to her last Story Hour where the *Owl Moon* filmstrip was shown (Weston Woods). Even though she was no longer able to talk, she indicated to her mother that she wanted a copy of the book. Shortly thereafter, her mother recounted that she had read the book three times to her child. Certain books in the pediatric library collection will have a transcendence that touches the reader and listener on many levels.

Building the core collection based on the preceding "quick references" and adding new titles where needed will result in a good collection for hospitalized children.

Chapter 3.

OFFERING A STORY HOUR FOR TODDLERS, PRESCHOOLERS, AND SIBLINGS

A few short years ago, three changes led to the development of hospital story hours for the very young child. The first was a shift in pediatric hospital populations. Infants through preschool age children began to represent 45% of the census. In a number of hospitals, very young children started flocking to story hours designed originally for ages 5 to 12.

Secondly, recent studies have shown that, between birth and age four, more intellectual development takes place than at any other time in a child's life.[1] It is important to address with stimulating and enriching materials this emerging ability to think, understand and express language, and to discern relationships. Hospital staff are concerned with the hospitalized child's growth and development. In this area, a librarian can offer a program that nurtures this crucial early developmental process.

Thirdly, in addressing the results of these studies, the American Library Association and local/regional public library systems have developed tested program materials that assure successful story hours in a variety of early childhood settings. These materials provide background information and programming that can also serve toddler/preschooler story hours in hospital settings.

GOALS

The goals of a Toddler/Preschooler Story Hour are to encourage verbalization, to introduce the child to the rhythm and flow of language, to enhance the child's abilities in group participation, and to promote positive parent/child interactions. The art of storytelling has its "own special niche in developing reflective thought, memory, and attention." [2]

HOSPITALIZED TODDLERS AND PRESCHOOLERS IN STORY HOUR

The young child may have had few group experiences. As a result, this age child may not participate readily. Specifically, the hospitalized young child may also be withdrawn due to possible parent/family separation, stranger anxiety, and unpleasant medical experiences.

While an ill child may have less energy than usual, she can be eager to move about as much as possible. Unexpectedly, this child may surge forward to the puppet stage, leaving the IV pole and line trailing precariously behind.

A child's arm may be secured with tape in order to hold the IV in place, but she will nearly always try to raise the flap in a lift-and-see picture book, reach for the book itself, or pat the soft mascot puppet. For unencumbered children, large movement story play is an opportunity for channeling energies, for experiencing a sense of accomplishment, and for feeling comfortable with their bodies and themselves.

The hospitalized toddler and preschooler will be particularly easily distracted. Concentration can be broken by another child's crying or the arrival of a parent — her own or someone else's — or the readjustment of an IV pump. The possibilities are endless.

LOCATION

Locating the Story Hour space on a floor where there is a large preschool population will minimize the often extraordinary efforts needed to move very young children along with IV poles and oxygen tanks onto elevators.

The room should have sufficient electrical outlets for a tape player, filmstrip projector, and necessary medical equipment.

In today's hospital space crunch, it can be a real challenge to find room for Story Hour. A high ratio of adults to children adds to the overcrowding. Maintain an open aisle to the door.

If Story Hour is located in a playroom, cover shelved toys with a sheet and move riding toys out of sight. This will help direct the child's attention to the storyteller. There will be enough other distractions for the young listener.

FORMAT

Late mornings seem best for Toddler Story Hours. Morning routines are usually completed and children are ready for play ac-

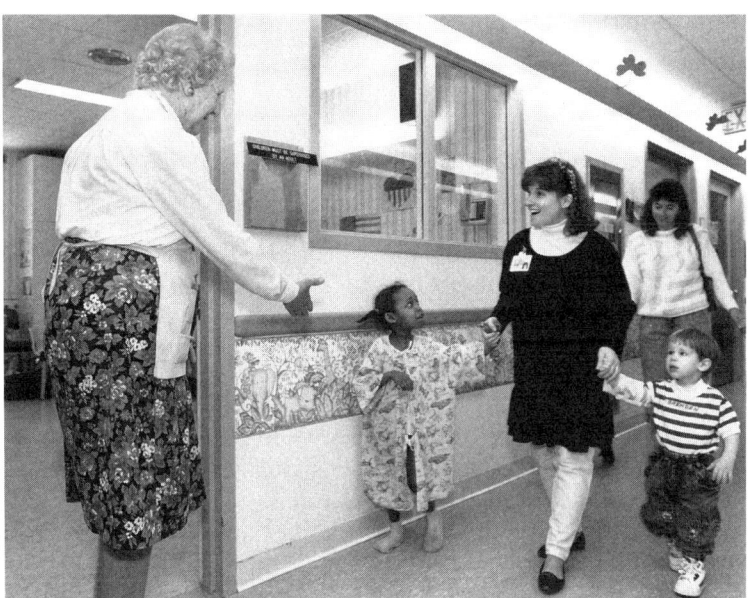

Arrival at Story Hour.

tivities. Frequently, parents must return to jobs and Story Hour can help fill the void created by their departures.

Because late arrivals are unavoidable, playing music or handling puppets can help pass time spent waiting for others who are on their way. A Story Hour apron for the librarian with pockets for small stuffed animals is good diversion, too.

GENERAL ELEMENTS OF STORY HOUR PROGRAMMING

"Children demand and need lots of pattern repetition."[3] Hospitalized young children respond to repetition. A "hello" and "goodbye" song used with the same melody and with almost identical words makes for a satisfying closure. The mascot puppet's appearance and then reappearance at program's end serves the same purpose.

The "Mascot" Story Hour Puppet:

Particularly in a hospital setting, the puppet acts as a non-threatening intermediary between the adult and the child. The puppet should be a warm and familiar object, e.g., a teddy bear or a bunny. Odd looking puppets add to the child's sense of unfamiliarity.

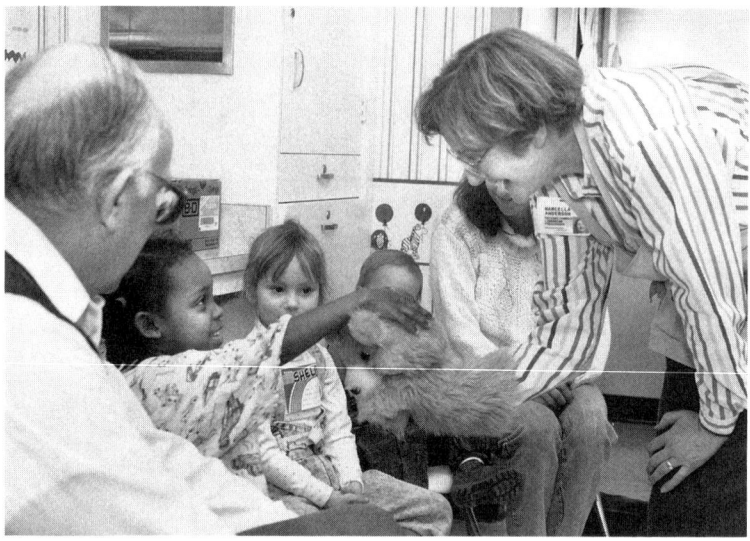

"Hello" to the teddy puppet mascot.

It is important not to thrust the puppet at the child, but to hold it at a distance. Adults may be encouraged to pat the puppet if the child seems reluctant or turns away. Often at the end of Story Hour, the reluctant child will smile, say "bye" or pat the puppet — a good indication that the child has been reassured and relaxed.

Music:

Nearly all young children enjoy music, and hospitalized preschoolers are no exception. Often immobilized in one way or another, they welcome the chance to shake, tap, or ring musical instruments. Chime bells on a fabric strip work best for tiny hands. Older preschoolers like the challenge of handbells and tambourines. Well-chosen cassette music or adult accompaniment on an Autoharp or piano add a pleasurable background and encourage participation. Upbeat melody and rhythm such as "Raindrops Keep Falling on My Head" (Bacharach) and quiet songs like "One Light, One Sun" (Raffi) after an active story hour ensure a positive conclusion.

Finger and Hand Play:

Parents, staff, and volunteers should take part in finger and hand plays. This encourages the children to participate. Often the children will simply watch adults the first time around. Action songs are especially popular; the music itself encourages participation.

Clap often in a hospital Story Hour — clap for the children and the children will clap for themselves. The young patient needs and appreciates this reaffirmation.

Flannel Board Stories:

Flannel board stories are big attention-getters. Even the most inattentive child will easily focus on the flannel board. "...A flannel board is the backbone of a successful toddler storytime." During and after Story Hour, the various figures "can be touched, held, and moved, forming a bridge between reality and the abstract." [4]

While educational supply stores and catalogs offer pre-made flannel board stories, it is also possible to create one's own, particularly for a story that has special meaning for the hospitalized child. The concrete images found in children's poetry lend themselves to flannel board presentation too. Very short stories found in children's magazines can also be adapted with appropriate credit to the author.

The public library has many helpful instruction books on making flannel board stories. (See Resources.)

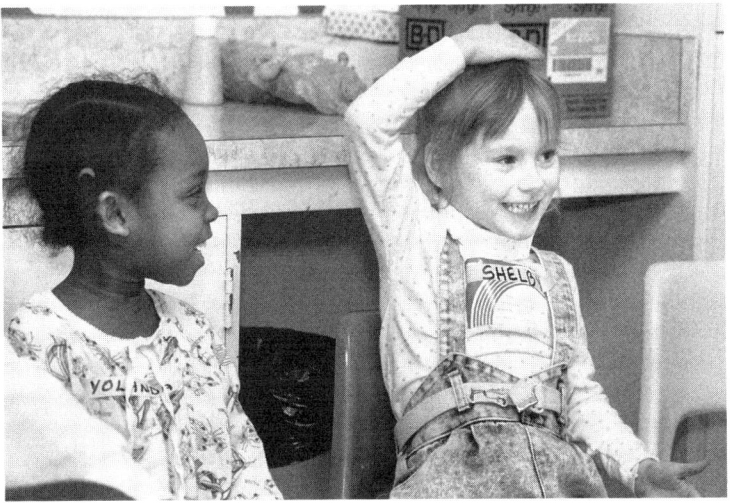

"Dress the teddy" time.

Puppet Shows:
Folklore appropriate for the young child can be presented through puppetry as another medium for storytelling and as a method of familiarizing children with their cultural literary heritage. In a hospital setting, it is advisable that the puppeteer relate her own narration rather than rely on a prepared cassette tape, especially in stories where chases and bangings around can be prolonged — to the excited delight of the older child, but to the distress of the hospitalized toddler beset already by fears and strangers. Professional puppeteers watch carefully through their scrim curtains and often preassess the audience, making adjustments they deem necessary. One puppeteer, sighting a seated child who was bald from chemotherapy, decided to drop a wild haircutting sequence that left the puppet with no hair.

Books:
Happily, books for the very young are abundant and the task is not so much to find a book as to choose one of high quality. In addition to new entries in this publishing field, old favorites are frequently republished, sometimes in paperback for the first time and sometimes with new, brighter, and updated illustrations and text.

The hospitalized toddler and preschooler need clear colors to attract and hold their attention. The librarian should know the story well enough so as not to fragment short attention spans by having to refer to the book herself. Be prepared to carry the book from child to child, eliciting his interest on an almost one-on-one basis.

Offer two books, perhaps three, depending on the group. Prepare the stories carefully.

Most public library preschool story hour programs begin with a finger or hand play. In a hospital setting, beginning with a book instead gives the child a chance to acclimate himself and catch his breath. He needs the moment to sit quietly.

For your first book, choose one with a strong and straightforward story line that offers an opportunity to "catch up" on the story for children arriving late. Young listeners like repetition and may even enjoy hearing the beginning again. Predictable books with repetitive phrases and cumulative sequence are especially recommended.

The second book may be one which calls for some interaction. By this time, the hospitalized child is more ready for participation.

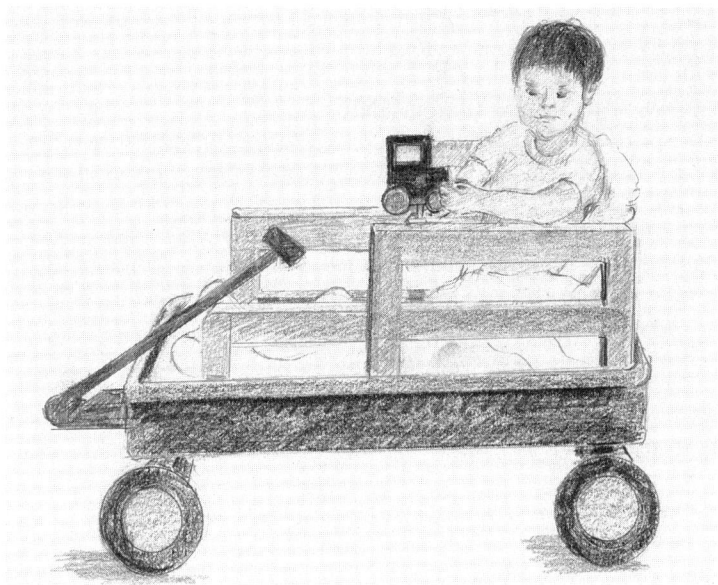

Play with a train engine Take-Away.

Take-Aways:

Story Hour listeners are usually eager to receive Take-Aways to help them remember a good time. Sometimes these are only partially completed creative projects. The children can plant the seed, color the picture in the Story Hour area or back in their playrooms, or frost and decorate the baked cookies.

Parents are also happy with Take-Aways. Very young parents are often seen in pediatric settings. Handouts can contribute to supporting parenting skills. Sometimes the material is a copy of the hand play or a short list of books used often in Story Hour. Two appealing brochures, "Raising a Young Reader" and "Learning Begins at Home," are always well received. (See Resources.) The librarian should recognize this opportunity to support the cause of effective parenting. In addition, some of these young parents are hearing stories of childhood for the very first time.

THE CHILD WHO MISSED STORY HOUR

The child whose treatment precluded Story Hour by a few minutes deserves a chance to experience a part of it. Show willingness to offer the child a chance to see the puppet show, flannel board story, or filmstrip. Often this diversion is exactly what the child needs following a medical treatment.

BEFORE AND AFTER TREATMENT

For the child who may not eat or drink for hours prior to certain procedures, Story Hour can help to pass the time and to occupy the child's mind.

The child who comes to Story Hour after disagreeable treatments sometimes relaxes to the point of sleeping during the program. Consider this a compliment.

Toddler/Preschooler Story Hour can affirm the parent as much as the child. Said one mother as she left, "I loved it as much as my three-year-old — maybe even more."

Chapter 4.

STORY HOUR PROGRAMMING FOR TODDLERS, PRESCHOOLERS, AND SIBLINGS

ATTENTION-GETTERS

In preparing the following programs, these attention-getters help to attract and hold the young child's interest.

Encourage children — and the adults — to join in making any sounds that are part of a story, e.g., the wind howled.

Props work well too. Preschoolers focus eyes and attention on a related object held by the person telling the story, such as an overall-clad teddy bear during *Corduroy* and *A Pocket for Corduroy* (Freeman). Occasionally, publishers sell stuffed characters from their books. While these visual aids are not inexpensive, owning at least one is a good investment for Toddler/Preschooler Story Hour.

Certain books are perfect vehicles for group participation. During the telling of *Martin's Hats* (Blos), one can add or omit kinds of hats as long as one stays true to the intent of the story and to its beginning and end.

Toddlers and preschoolers take pride in learning many new skills. Dressing themselves is one skill that may be "lost" during hospitalization. Children sitting before you in hospital gowns, slippers, and robes achieve a sense of mastery during the fun of correcting a teddy bear who dresses himself backwards.

Older visiting siblings serve as enthusiastic role models for Story Hour participation.

PROGRAMS

1.   On the Farm

Books: *The Big Sneeze* (Brown, R.)
Spot Goes to the Farm (Hill)
The Big, Red Barn (Brown, M.W.)
Hattie and the Fox (Fox)
Pumpkin, Pumpkin (Titherington)

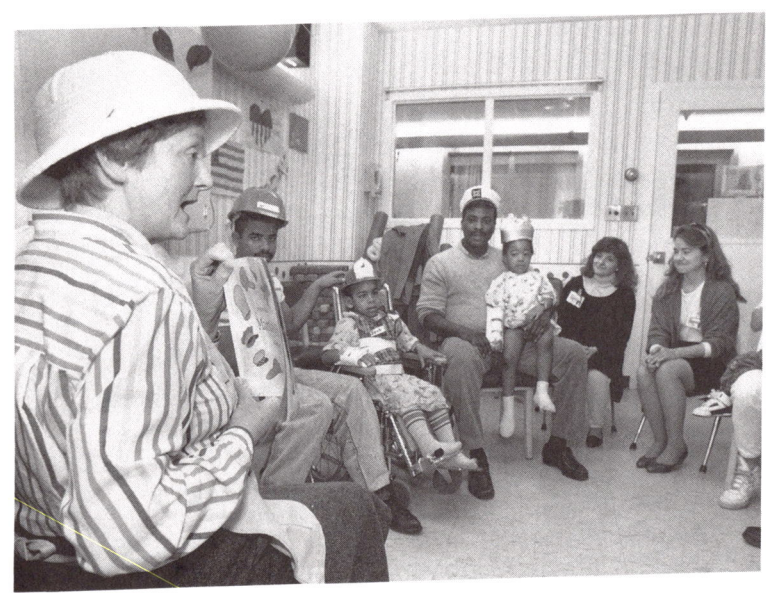

Participation in listening to Martin's Hats.

Finger/   Pancake — *Clap Your Hands* (Hayes)
Hand Play: Five Fat Peas — *Clap Your Hands* (Hayes)

Flannel Board: *The Turnip* (Domanska)
               The Three Pigs

Puppetry: Old MacDonald Had a Farm
          Little Red Hen
          The Gingerbread Boy

Filmstrip: *The Midnight Farm* (Lindbergh), *Rosie's Walk* (Hutchins)

Activity/Take-Away: Decorate baked gingerbread boy cookies.
                 Make stick puppets of gingerbread boy, then
                 attach cut-out figure to a drinking straw.

2.   Fliers, Crawlers, and Jumpers

Books: *The Very Hungry Caterpillar* (Carle)
          The Very Busy Spider (Carle)
          The Very Quiet Cricket (Carle)
          The Bee (Ernst)

Finger/   Incey Wincey Spider — *Clap Your Hands* (Hayes)
Hand Play: The Caterpillar — *Hand Rhymes* (Brown, M.)

Flannel Board: *The Very Hungry Caterpillar* (Carle)

Activity/Take-Away: Make a tissue paper butterfly.
                            Cut out a caterpillar-shape bookmark.

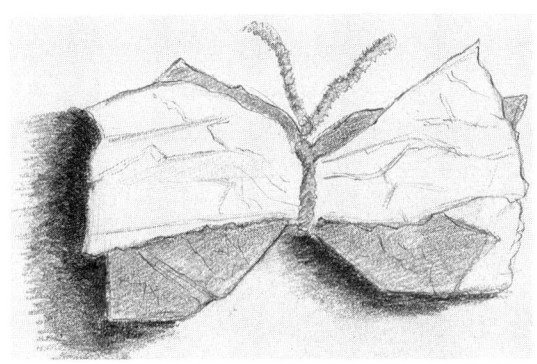

3.   Bears, Bears, Everywhere!

Books: *Are You There, Bear?* (Maris)
              Corduroy and *A Pocket for Corduroy* (Freeman)
              My Brown Bear Barney (Butler)
              Brown Bear, Brown Bear, What Do You See? (Martin, B.)

Finger/   Going on a Bear Hunt — *Storytimes for*
Hand Play: *Two-Year-Olds* (Nichols)
                Dress the Teddy — *How Do I Put It On?* (Watanabe)

Flannel Board: Ten in the Bed
                The Three Bears

Activity/Take-Away: Put teddy bear stickers on a bookmark.
                            Photocopy illustrations for coloring
                            (give illustrator credit).

4.   Trains, Buses, Boats

Books: *The Wheels on the Bus* (Kovalski)
              Mr. Little's Noisy Car (Fowler)
              The Little Engine That Could (Piper)
              Four Brave Sailors (Ginsburg)

Finger/   Here Comes the Choo-choo Train — *Let's Do*
Hand Play: *Fingerplays* (Grayson)
               Meet the Boats — *Storytimes for Two-Year-Olds*
               (Nichols)

Flannel Board: *Mr. Gumpy's Outing* (Burningham)

Activity/Take-Away: Make train engine puppets. Glue on details of
               paper engine, then attach to a drinking straw.
               Make sailboats from foil with paper sails.

5.   Frogs, Turtles, Rabbits, Birds

Books: *Jump, Frog, Jump!* (Kalan)
               The Tale of Peter Rabbit (Potter)
               My Spring Robin (Rockwell)
               Home for a Bunny (Brown)

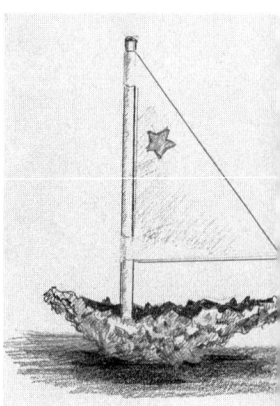

Finger/   I Had a Little Turtle —
Hand Play: *Clap Your Hands* (Hayes)
               Bunny — *Finger*
               Frolics (Cromwell)

Puppetry: The Tortoise and the Hare

Filmstrip: *Are You My Mother?* (Eastman)
           The Runaway Bunny (Brown, M.W.)

Activity/Take-Away: Make a paper frog or rabbit puppet. Cut out,
               then attach to a drinking straw.
               Photocopy an illustrated poem to color
               (give credits).

6.   About Me All Year

Books: *It's Just Me, Emily* (Hines)
               Martin's Hats (Blos)
               If I Were a Penguin... (Goennel)
               Goodbye, House (Asch)
               Shhhh (Henkes)
               Not a Little Monkey (Zolotow)

Finger/   I Have a Nose — *Storytimes for Two-Year-Olds*
               (Nichols)

Hand Play: My Book — *Hand Rhymes* (Brown, M.)
                    How Do I Put It On? (Watanabe)
                    Ten Little Fingers — *Finger Frolics* (Cromwell)

Flannel Board: *Just Like Me* (Ormerod)

Filmstrip: *I Like Me* (Carlson)
                Umbrella (Yashima)

Activity/Take-Away: Take a Polaroid
    photo of each child. Mount
    on color construction paper.
    Draw around child's hand —
    write name and date.
    Use washable markers.

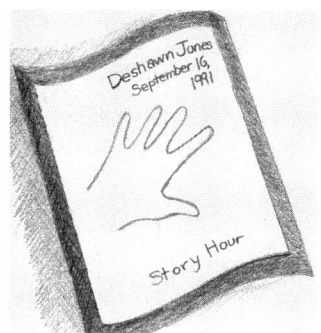

a. In Summer:

Books   *A Summer Day* (Florian)
                For Strawberry Jam or Fireflies (Hartman)

Finger/
Hand Play: Bees — *Finger Frolics* (Cromwell)

Filmstrip: *Titch* (Hutchins)

Activity/Take-Away: Draw an imagined plant from a dried bean glued
                        to bottom of paper.

b. In Fall:

Books: *Pumpkin, Pumpkin* (Titherington)
                Anna's Rain (Burstein)

Finger/
Hand Play: In the Apple Tree — *Finger Frolics* (Cromwell)

Activity/Take-Away: Paste colored leaves on bare, paper tree.

c. In Winter:

Books: *Something Is Going to Happen* (Zolotow)
                The Mitten (Brett)

c. In Winter, continued:

Finger/
Hand Play: Chubby Little Snowman — *Finger Frolics* (Cromwell)

Activity/Take-Away: Begin a construction paper snowman for children to finish.

d. In Spring:

Books: *My Spring Robin* (Rockwell)
         Mother's Day Mice (Bunting)

Finger/
Hand Play: I Dig, Dig, Dig — *Storytimes for Two-Year-Olds* (Nichols)

Filmstrip: *Picnic* (McCully)

Activity/Take-Away: Plant beans or peas in cups with small drain holes.

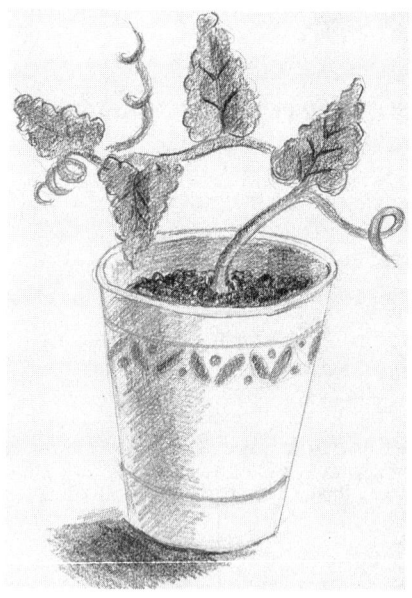

Careful planning offers the best opportunity for a meaningful and fun Story Hour. Success is sometimes simply hearing a three-year-old say to a nurse entering unexpectedly: "We don't like to be disturbed," or noting a child life specialist's remark: "In Story Hour for the little ones, everybody wins."

Chapter 5.

OFFERING A STORY HOUR FOR SCHOOL AGE CHILDREN AND SIBLINGS

Nearly everyone likes stories; much of what we communicate is through stories. Children especially "learn to use the content of stories to organize what they encounter of the world."[1] In a pediatric setting, Story Hour tries to encourage the creative imagination in all the children, providing them with a chance to escape from the realities of medical procedures and the stress of hospitalization. Storytelling in hospitals is grounded in the belief that "stories are as essential to our lives as food and water, as sleep, dreams and love."[2]

AUDIENCE CONSIDERATIONS

Mastery experienced vicariously through a story can carry over to mastering the difficulties of hospitalization — hard feelings, pain, and the medical environment. School age children respond particularly well to these possibilities.

Nearly all school age children's feelings for other patients are sensitized in and out of Story Hour and are often expressed by the request for a Story Hour Take-Away to give to a friend who couldn't come. Be prepared with enough Take-Aways so this is possible.

Hospitalized children are not eager to leave Story Hour. After thirty to forty minutes in a "safe," appealing place, they are relaxed. They have enjoyed a change from the hospital room, respite from medical regimen, and some happy and exciting moments. They have been with other children in an atmosphere that is familiar and pleasurable. Often they are in a "state of altered consciousness," a kind of hypnosis as a result of storytelling.[3] Frequently, stress levels are lowered and an environment has been offered where healing may start to take place. These are important goals of Story Hour.

A child may take from Story Hour just one new concept, one new character to read about, one new understanding, or one new fact to pursue. Finally, he will carry with him the certainty that he is cared about and respected. That he is important to the librarian helps to affirm his belief in his own self-worth at a time of personal vulnerability.

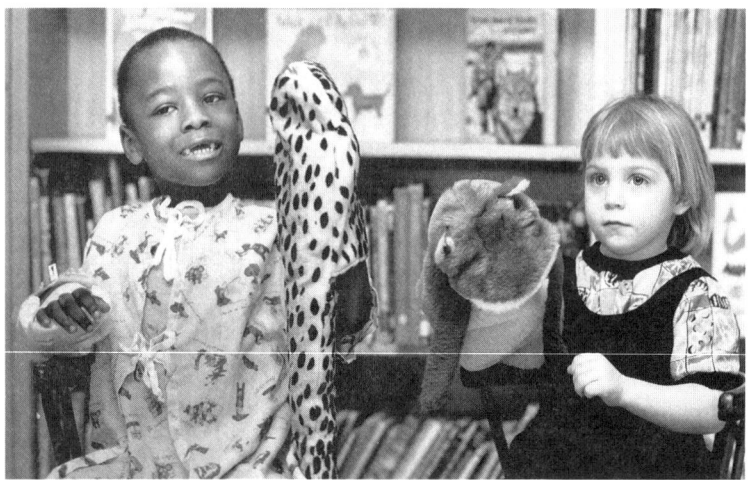

Children use puppets to help the librarian tell the story.

PROGRAM CONSIDERATIONS

A School Age Story Hour attracts a wide age range from five to fourteen. Preparing at least six picture books for various age levels averts panic when mostly young children arrive or the gathered group is predominantly older. If the group is young, include a flannel board story or a reliable favorite like *The Very Hungry Caterpillar* (Carle). If restlessness occurs, introduce finger/hand play. Should an older group arrive, a book like *Aurora Means Dawn* (Sanders) is a good choice. Today, many picture books have themes that are appropriate for the older listener.

The school age child enjoys puppetry and is eager to participate in a performance. Most often, children take part from where they are seated. Usually, visiting siblings prefer to stand at the front of the room and face the group.

It is a good idea also to have more than one filmstrip at hand; usually children wait patiently as changes are made.

Flexibility in the choice of materials enables one to relate to as many children as possible.

THE ENVIRONMENT

Be prepared for the unexpected. Paper towels, tissues, latex gloves, and antibacterial soap are good supplies to have on hand. No medical treatments or even cursory examinations of a child should be permitted during Story Hour.

Consider general safety during Story Hour. IV pump cords can be hazardous. If oxygen is in use, do not light birthday candles.

Anticipation of interruptions helps one to accept them as they occur. Children may be taken out for tests, a beeping IV pump may need adjustment, a child may suddenly cry or become ill. Depend on the other adults to help out so that the story can be continued — or pause until the situation has been tended to, then continue with a brief recap.

Always assure that other adults are present. Ask that at least one child life specialist remain in attendance.

Certain interruptions can be controlled. The phone can be answered by a volunteer; the intercom should be turned off, except for the librarian's use to call out in an emergency. A "Story Hour in Progress" sign on the closed front door reinforces the request to enter quietly and can direct late arrivals to an entrance at the rear of the room. A cardboard clock with moveable hands indicates Story Hour's duration.

When arranging chairs, leave a center aisle open to use in case of an emergency.

Support the adult who decides to remove a disruptive child. Perhaps that child would be better served in a one-on-one situation.

The disappointed child who has arrived too late for Story Hour should, like the toddler/preschooler, be given the opportunity to see the filmstrip and select books to take back to her room.

PLANNING AHEAD

All Story Hours benefit from a theme. When themes have been decided upon, start early to gather materials from the hospital library collection or from the public library, particularly for holiday themes. Some materials may have to be ordered or substitutions made.

BOOK SELECTION

The librarian should plan on presenting three books. The first book for the younger listeners is not necessarily theme-related. Usually, it is one where the story line will not suffer from interruptions of late arrivals and is frequently one that encourages group participation. Sometimes, after the first story, younger children will want to leave because of their short attention spans.

The second book is also not necessarily theme-related. Usually, it is one with emotional overtones, often a story about changes in the family: new home, new baby, divorce, remarriage, job loss and hard times. Finding herself in a personally difficult situation may heighten the child's response to the problem-related story and to the identifiable character's efforts in problem or attitude resolution.

The third selection introduces the theme and related artifacts, maps, photos, filmstrip, activity, and a take-away — an enhancement or reminder of Story Hour.

PREPARATION ON THE PATIENT FLOORS

Assuming that an advance schedule of programming has been given to the various floors, an early phone call on Story Hour day to the child life specialist on each floor reminds her of Story Hour's theme or event. This information aids her in publicizing Story Hour. At the same time, the librarian can be apprised of several details: the expected size of the group from a specific floor, the child with a sensory impairment who may come, children who cannot take food, and the number of patients arriving in beds.

The children are brought by child life specialists, volunteers, parents/grandparents, teachers, and student nurses. Encourage the child life specialists to send the children with name tags so that they can be greeted by name and be called upon by name as Story Hour progresses. Have adhesive tape and pen ready for those who arrive without name tags.

A few hospitals like Minneapolis Children's Medical Center, MN, provide closed circuit television viewings of Story Hours for children who cannot leave their rooms. At Cook-Fort Worth Children's Medical Center, TX, a volunteer is at the child's bedside to help with the follow-up craft project.

THE GROUP GATHERS

It is important to greet each child warmly without being overwhelming. Arrange to be free to give some special attention to the early arrivals who may wait five or ten minutes for the group to gather. This is a good time for one-on-one reading and for individual help with book selection. Volunteers are of particular assistance here.

Children may be afraid of a child with an abnormal appearance and refuse to sit near him. Place an adult next to that child so that he does not, under any circumstances, sit alone.

It is difficult for everyone to see seriously ill or disabled children come into Story Hour. Adults who work with hospitalized children learn to look beyond the conditions of serious disability and illness, beneath the bandages and casts, to find the child within.

Certain children may ask: "What's wrong with her?" It is enough to answer simply in a general way with emphasis on recovery: "I think that she is feeling better now that she's able to come to Story Hour."

TIME TO START

As in the Story Hour for the younger children, introduce an "ice breaker." Our fluffy mascot dog puppet, "Winston," is a well-loved fixture of School Age Story Hour. Many children remember him from earlier hospitalizations and some greet him with a hand in his toothless mouth. To the children's delight, "Winston" recites poetry along with the librarian.

Under stress of hospitalization, some children fear they will lose their self-control. It is important that the librarian present herself as a person who is in charge and one who will be in control of any unforeseen event. A structured, well-planned program gives confidence to the librarian that carries over to her listeners.

Hospitalized children can come into Story Hour in various states. They may be worried, frightened, sleepy, lonely, feeling ill, uncomfortable, angry, or enervated. They may also come feeling eager, energized, and ready for a good time. The former group is the special challenge. In a hospital Story Hour, the storyteller must be creative in thinking of ways to capture the child's interest in the "story web."

THE STORY

The following is an example of ways to use visual aids and to subtly dramatize the action as in *William Tell* (Bawden). Before starting the story, hold up a poster board with the names of the three sections (cantons) that make up present-day Switzerland. With an apple, dramatize the Bailiff Gessler's challenge to Tell to shoot the apple off the head of Tell's young son. When Gessler's men search the mountains for the escaped Tell, interject an echo dialog:

"WILLIAM TELL — William Tell" two or three times. At story's end, hold up a poster board with the name "Switzerland" and a large color scene of the country. Show Switzerland on a world map.

Sometimes slow-moving sections of a story or parts that are threatening to the hospitalized child can be abridged "while preserving the original words, the characteristic phrases and the sentence structure."[4]

Where conversation is merely described, consider transposing it into direct dialog for more liveliness.

Know well the beginning and ending so as to be true to the author's style and the aptly chosen words. Memorize the repetitions to use them verbatim. While repetition is essential to a picture book's structure, it is also an enthusiastic way for children to participate. Like all children, young patients enjoy the participation. As in all story hours, some groups are more responsive than others.

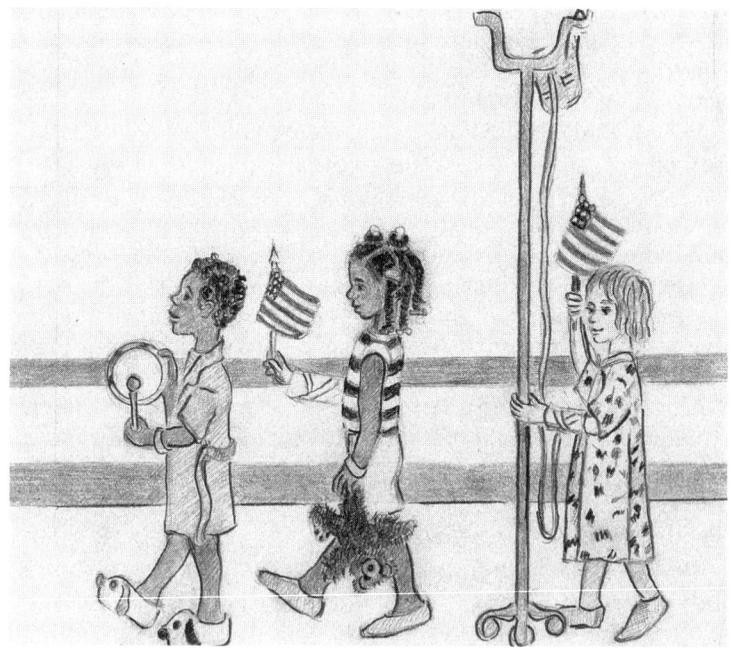

Fourth of July Story Hour Parade.

When the story is over, it's simply over. No additional comments are required. "A good story is sufficient unto the day. It is complete as it stands. If it has something to teach, let it teach in its own sufficiency. Let it keep its magic and fulfill its purpose. In other words, let it be."[5]

FOLLOW-UP ACTIVITY

A planned follow-up activity can introduce a festive sense of closure. Story Hour parades for President's Day and the Fourth of July are enthusiastically received by spectators and participants. Said one father as he marched past the librarian, "Gramma will never believe this!" Another time, a parent was overhead saying to her husband: "Put on your shoes, Raymond. We're going to be in a parade!"

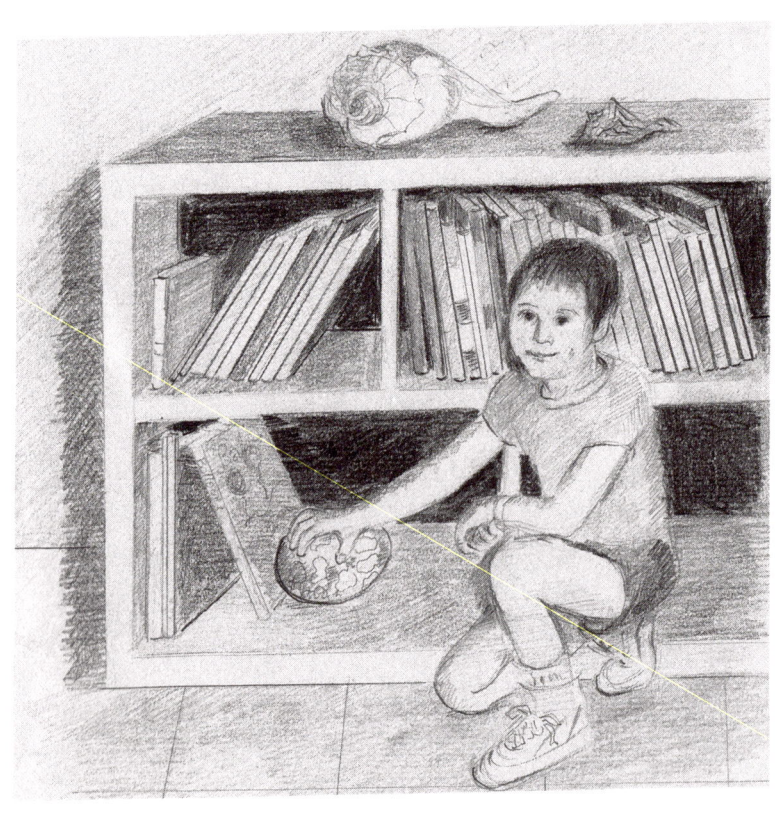

A child finds the "dinosaur egg."

Chapter 6.

STORY HOUR PROGRAMMING FOR SCHOOL AGE CHILDREN AND SIBLINGS

This chapter introduces seven popular, "hospital-tested" themes. Over time, librarians develop their own favorites. Often, they are themes with particular pertinence to the location of the hospital and local history.

PROGRAMS

1.   Dinosaurs

Books: *Patrick's Dinosaurs* (Carrick)
             What Happened to Patrick's Dinosaurs? (Carrick)
             There's No Such Thing as a Dragon (Kent)
             Tyrannosaurus Was a Beast (Prelutsky)
             Bones, Bones, Dinosaur Bones (Barton)
             Dinosaurs (Gibbons)

Filmstrip: *The Mysterious Tadpole* (Kellogg)
             Danny and the Dinosaur (Hoff)

Activity: Find a dinosaur egg in the library (mark a honeydew
             melon with spots and circles).
             Following guides in Gibbons, cut out paper dinosaur
             footprints; measure out length of stride and head
             height of largest dinosaur for children to visualize.

Take-Away: Store bought or homemade dinosaur cookies.
             Dinosaur stickers on a bookmark

2.   Friends Everywhere

Books: *The Day of Ahmed's Secret* (Heide) — Egypt
             William Tell (Bawden) — Switzerland

Thunder Cake (Polacco) — Russia
Not So Fast, Songololo (Daly) — South Africa
Tiki, Tiki Tembo (Mosel) — China
The First Rains (Bonnici) — East India

Filmstrip: *Strega Nona* (dePaola) — Italy
Here Comes the Cat (Asch) — Russia

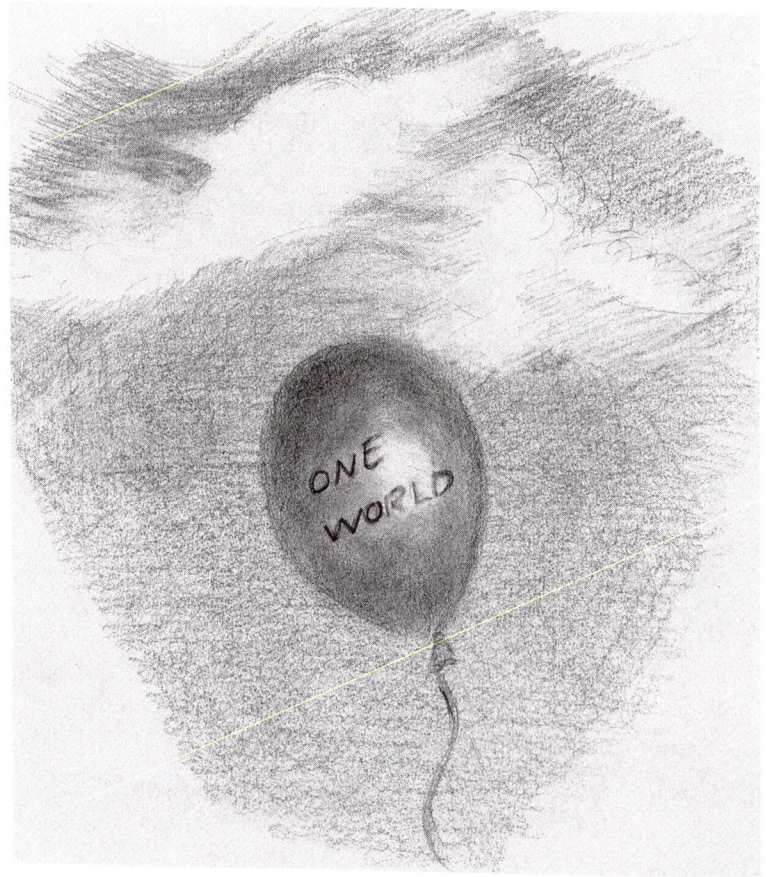

Activity: Serve spaghetti, or a cake similar to that baked in *Thunder Cake*.
Send up a balloon labeled "One World."

3.   Our Earth, Sea, And Sky

Books: *Hey, Get Off Our Train* (Burningham)
           What is Beyond the Hill? (Ekker)
           The Owl and the Woodpecker (Wildesmith)
           Fireflies (Brinckloe)
           The Lost Lake (Say)
           Come a Tide (Lyon)
           Anna's Garden Songs (Steele) — poetry
           The Old Ladies Who Liked Cats (Greene)
           How Many Stars in the Sky? (Hort)

Filmstrip: *Owl Moon* (Yolen)
           A Tree is Nice (Udry)

Activity: Plant peas or beans in paper cups with drain holes.

Take-Away: Give out shells or interesting stones.
           Hand out list of things to do to "make every day
           Earth Day."

4.   Native Americans

Books: *Good Hunting, Blue Sky* (Parish)
           The Fire Bringer (Hodges) — Beat on a drum while tell-
           ing about the race from the fire spirits.
           The Legend of the Indian Paintbrush (dePaola)
           The Star Maiden (Esbensen)
           Dancing Tepees — Indian poetry
           Knots on a Counting Rope (Martin, B. and Archambault)

Filmstrip: *Arrow to the Sun* (McDermott)

Activity: Teach a few Indian words or phrases in Indian sign
           language.

Take-Away: Popcorn made in Story Hour

5.   Adventurers

Books: *Androcles and the Lion* (Galdone)
           Henry Explores the Mountains (Taylor)
           Lost in the Storm (Carrick)
           Aurora Means Dawn (Sanders)

> *Brave Irene* (Steig) — omit reference to
> giving up and dying

Filmstrip: *Snuff* (Blake)
            The Day Jimmy's Boa ate the Wash (Kellogg)

Activity: Have child write own initials on explorer flag taped to
            a straw.

Take-Away: Hero medals — gold notary seal attached to ribbon
            to stick onto child's clothing

6.   Families

Books: *Tight Times* (Hazen)
            My Mother's Getting Married Again (Drescher)
            Christina Katerina and the Great Bear Train (Gauch)
            Jamaica Tag-Along (Havill)
            Grandma's Baseball (Curtis)
            Amifika (Clifton)
            A Beautiful Sea Shell (Bornstein)

Filmstrip: *Picnic* (McCully)
            Aunt Nina and Her Nephews and Nieces (Brandenberg)

Take-Away: A flower to give to a family member

7.   Holidays and Special Events

a. Black History Month

Books: *Grampa's Face* (Greenfield)
            Flossie and the Fox (McKissack)

Poetry: "Dreams" (Hughes) — *Don't You Turn Back* (Hughes)

b. Valentine's Day

Books: *The Valentine Bears* (Bunting)
          One Zillion Valentines (Modell)

Poetry: "Love" (Silverstein) — *Where the Sidewalk Ends*
          (Silverstein)

c. St. Patrick's Day

Books: *St. Patrick's Day in the Morning* (Bunting)
          The Field of Buttercups (Boden)

Poetry: "The Little Elf" (Bangs) — *All the Silver Pennies*
          (Thompson, sel.)

d. Easter/Passover

Books: *Tico and the Golden Wings* (Lionni)
          A Rabbit for Easter (Carrick)
          Could Anything Be Worse? (Hirsh) — Set story at Passover
             time.

Poetry: "April" (Teasdale) — *Collected Poems* (Teasdale)

e. For Mothers and Other Caregivers

Books: *The Mother's Day Mice* (Bunting)
          I'm Telling You Now (Delton)

Poetry: "I Hear My Mother's..." (Whitman), "New Mother"
          (Marks) [stepparent] — *Poems for Mothers* (Livingston, sel.)

f. For Fathers and Other Caregivers

Books: *No Nap* (Bunting)
          My Dad the Magnificent (Parker)

Poetry: "Daddy Fell into the Pond" (Noyes), "My Jose" (Robin-
          son) [stepparent] — *Poems for Fathers* (Livingston, sel.)

g. Fourth of July

Books: *Andy and the Lion* (Daugherty) — The parade finale can be
             a Fourth of July parade.
          The Hokey-Pokey Man (Kroll)

Poetry: "Fourth of July Night" (Aldis) — *Poetry for Holidays*
          (Larrick, sel.)

h. Halloween

Books: *Miss Nelson is Missing* (Allard)
        A Tiger Called Thomas (Zolotow)
Poetry: "Pumpkin Head" (Fisher)—*Out in the Dark and Daylight* (Fisher)

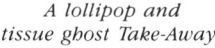

A lollipop and tissue ghost Take-Away.

i. Thanksgiving

Books: *Can I Help?* (Rockwell)
        How Many Days to America? (Bunting)
Poetry: "Giving Thanks" (Merriam)
        — *Thanksgiving Poems* (Livingston, sel.)

j. Christmas/Hanukkah

Books: *The Silver Christmas Tree* (Hutchins)
        The Shepherd Boy (Lewis)
        Latkes and Applesauce (Manushkin)

Poetry: "December" (Fisher) — *Out in the Dark and Daylight* (Fisher)

A FEW AFTERTHOUGHTS

In recognition of Children's Book Week, Right to Read Week, and National Library Week, special story hours are recommended:

Books: *The Wednesday Surprise* (Bunting)
        When Will I Read? (Cohen)
        The Day of Ahmed's Secret (Heide)

Poetry: "Keep a Poem in Your Pocket" (de Regniers)
        "Poetry" (Farjeon)
        "Things" (Greenfield)

Take-Away: Plastic book bags, pins, pencils, or bookmarks (See Resources).

Hospitalized children can feel less isolated knowing that from the hospital they are joining their schoolmates in celebrating these special weeks.

Keep in mind that certain books are Story Hour classics and can be used with almost any theme. Your children's librarian at the public library can recommend titles for you — ask about responses when she used them herself.

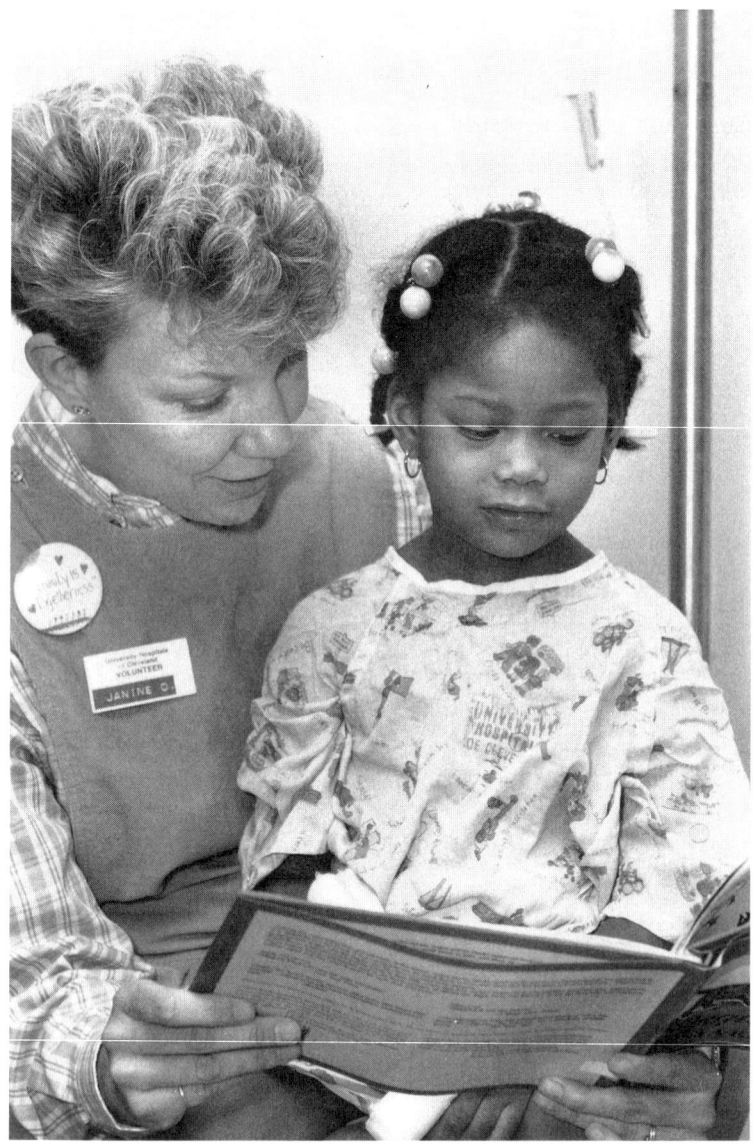

Chapter 7.

READING ALOUD TO THE HOSPITALIZED CHILD

One of the most important aspects of reading aloud to the hospitalized child is his knowledge that someone who cares about him is near — someone who cares enough about him to share a book.

A six-year-old frequently hospitalized child with a serious lung disorder was admitted to the intensive care unit and received treatment to relieve his severe difficulty with breathing.

Soon thereafter, a child life specialist went to his bed with an assortment of books to read aloud to him. From a number of titles well known to this child, he chose *The Little Engine That Could* (Piper), a story familiar to him from home.

When the child life specialist first arrived, the child was coughing and agitated from the tube that was placed in his throat. At length, listening to a story that reminded him of home and reinforced a search for hope, he closed his eyes and rested.

Hospitalized children who are read aloud to do not stare vacantly at the TV nor lie isolated with empty minds. Rather, the stories they have heard can become the stuff of their thinking. They can also tell and retell the stories within their own heads.

Reading aloud to all kinds of listeners is a general practice in pediatric settings. In recent years, the practice has been more emphasized in our hospital and more often scheduled into a pediatric therapy program.

The person — librarian, volunteer, child life specialist — who reads aloud to the hospitalized child will find the following guidelines helpful. Take the time to refer to Chapter 2 for developmental stages, concerns of the hospitalized child, and appropriate book titles. Some hospitals develop special collections of books for reading aloud.

GOALS FOR READING ALOUD

1. Enhancement of the child's sense that he is cared about.
2. Comfort, pleasure, and relaxation through quiet voice tones and language that flows and sometimes rhymes.

3. Imaginative separation from a stressful situation, an escape from boredom.

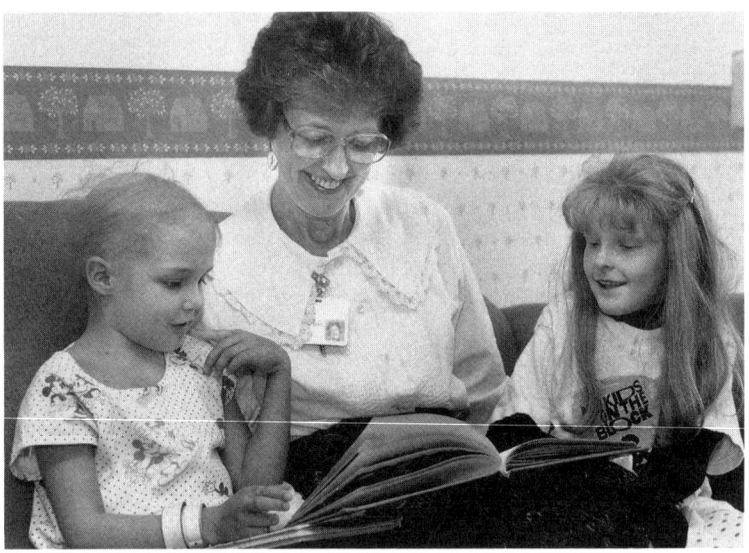

Young patients and a child life specialist enjoy a "read-along" in the lounge.

PREPARATION FOR READING ALOUD

A staff member who knows the patients and their situations can identify which child would benefit from a reading aloud time. Sometimes, this child is withdrawn, in pain, anxious, depressed, or lonely. Occasionally, the child is premedicated and awaiting surgery or treatment.

In selecting books, it is important to remember that ill and injured children have short attention spans. Choose materials that have high interest levels and are not overly lengthy. Some books for older readers have chapters that are both brief and self-contained.

It is a good idea to have several books at the appropriate level for the child. If she is old enough, making her own choices provides desirable interaction and a chance for her to be in control.

Younger children will simply enjoy appropriate picture books, but may need additional inducement to pay attention. Pop-up, half-page, and lift-the-flap books are much enjoyed. Flannel board stories are popular and puppets elicit easy responses, even from the child who seems withdrawn. Children will interact with both these mediums.

Inquire as to the reading interests of the older school age patient. This information comes from the parent or child. Then, briefly review each book to become familiar with the contents. Some books may have segments that are threatening to a child who is already feeling vulnerable. Such segments may touch on the death of a minor character, burial of a pet, parental abandonment, or the end of a nurturing relationship with teacher, neighbor, or friend. Contemporary titles for the older school age child are often heavy on reality and address issues that can be overwhelming for the listener in an already difficult personal situation.

Hospitalized listeners of all ages may prefer books that are familiar. Sometimes a child will ask you to read a story that he might consider "babyish" under other circumstances, as behavioral regression is common during hospitalization.

PROCEDURES FOR READING ALOUD

Before starting to read, make an introductory remark like: "Do you know Mike Mulligan and his steam shovel? He's a special friend of mine." Or: "I bet you already know a lot about dinosaurs."

Be aware of the environment. Turn off the radio or TV. In some cases, closing the curtains around the bed helps to eliminate distractions.

Sit as close to the child as possible. Some children can sit in the reader's lap.

In simplifying or shortening the text, keep the story moving and never omit the repetition that is so important to the very young listener.

Read with expression, but SLOWLY so the child has time to process mental images of what he is hearing. It is difficult for the hospitalized child to concentrate.

Sometimes, the reader finds that roommates benefit from the reading aloud even more than the child indentified initially, as do visiting siblings and parents. Welcome their participation!

Some children are in no mood for conversation. One patient told a reader: "Another book, but no more talking."

If a child is NPO (nothing-by-mouth), he may not wish to hear a story about a birthday cake or picnics. Other patients may not be bothered by this aspect.

Occasionally, a child may want to read to you. He may say: "I'll read a page and you read a page" or he may simply turn the page at the appropriate time. This personal involvement helps to maintain alertness and interest.

If appropriate, show caring and concern for the child who wants to share her feelings with you. BE A GOOD LISTENER.

If the child drifts off, do not hurry from the room. He may be startled if he awakens and you are gone. In a very few minutes, he may open his eyes and be happy to see you still by his bed. This can be the start of a trusting relationship.

Interruptions are all too common and can be disconcerting to the person who is reading aloud. Sometimes, it helps to close the child's door and post on it a "Please Do Not Disturb" sign. A clock sign with moveable hands indicating the duration of the reading time will prevent a person opening the door with the inevitable query: "How long will you be?"

Keep in mind that medical treatments and the arrival of visitors cannot always be anticipated. It is hard not to become frustrated by the fact that medical procedures do take precedence over psychosocial support services. Other times, a medical procedure can wait. Clear communication with medical personnel is essential. Family and friends may offer to return shortly.

Be ready to share appropriately any responses to the literature that may be of interest to other staff members. After hearing *The Hole in the Dike* (Green), a child drank her first glass of water in three days.

If it seems appropriate, leave the book for the child or other persons to reread or continue reading, but emphasize where and how the book must be returned.

If you make a promise to return to a child's room, keep the promise. This is always important.

Sometimes, one wonders if a child has really heard a story. A child life specialist accompanied a young patient to a MRI scan. As the child lay in the tunnel, she sat behind the child's head and read *Peter Pan* (Barrie). It seemed the child was not listening, but the next week the child informed the child life specialist that all through her reading aloud, she had mispronounced an important word: "Neverland."

Show enthusiasm in your reading aloud, and your enthusiasm will be shared.

RESPONSES TO READING ALOUD

Some children need the playful persuasion of a friendly reader to agree to listen to books and stories. Responses are as varied as the children read to.

In general, though, the reader experiences a gratifying response to any efforts. The crying younger child usually stops sobbing and looks bug-eyed at puppets and lift-and-see books. A two-and-a-half-year-old having what her mother called "a grumpy day" smiled suddenly at the puppets and kissed them. A school age child in traction stopped sighing and grimacing as the reading progressed.

Sometimes, the reader experiences the results of a relationship quickly made. An asthmatic three-year-old refused to let an entering staff person make a mask exchange. Easily into a trust relationship with the reader, he allowed her to make the exchange.

An eight-year-old stabbing victim medicated prior to a dressing change asked the reader for "funny books" with an amusing character and chose *Amelia Bedelia* (Parish) and *Miss Nelson Is Missing* (Allard). Another time, a young burn patient asked the reader to stay and keep reading during painful physical therapy.

Reassured that their child is involved in a pleasant pastime, often parents will leave the room for a much-needed break. The parents of a six-year-old waiting to go to surgery were not present when the reader entered her room. When the reader finished *Mother's Day Mice* (Bunting), the child whispered conspiratorily in the reader's ear that Mother's Day was coming and did she know that?

A particularly hard situation may exist for a child injured in a car accident. A parent may also be injured and under treatment in a different hospital, therefore unable to visit. This circumstance creates fears and a poignant loneliness. The closeness and warmth of a read-aloud time with a caring adult helps to meet this child's special needs.

Sometimes, a reader is rebuffed one day and welcomed the next. If the child asks whether you will return and read some more, give an honest answer. Children who are angry and hostile are best served by being left some books for a later time.

A child who has not been sleeping well may drop into a deep slumber. The combination of a good story and a reassuring adult presence can make the difference.

Sometimes, simply sitting with a child — talking and sharing — can be as therapeutic as reading to him.

The experience and memory of being read to in a trying circumstance may nurture a developing lifelong love of books and reading.

"Smile when you enter the room," said a read-aloud volunteer. "Smile when you are reading, and smile when you say 'goodbye.'" Many children are happy to respond, thus reinforcing relaxation and pleasure.

Chapter 8.

LIBRARY SERVICES TO CHILDREN WITH SPECIAL NEEDS

Major pediatric hospitals serve the child with special needs requiring specialized medical skills and team management. At any given time, there are a number of young patients who can benefit from the various interventions offered by the library program.

Before selecting materials, it is important to understand the child's developmental and cognitive levels, regardless of her special needs. Discussion with a parent, child life specialist, nurse, or interaction with the child herself can help you to obtain this information.

The child's special needs will influence the librarian's approach. The following anecdotal vignettes illustrate specific needs, their impact on the child, and the adaptation in the use of library materials as informal interventions.

Janice — A Child with Hearing Impairment

A head nurse asked the librarian to visit this friendly young adolescent. Learning that she liked animals, the librarian took in carefully selected books for her enjoyment. Several were in the series *Books for World Explorers* published by The National Geographic Society. From a stack of other books, Janice chose *Hans Brinker or the Silver Skates* (Dodge), published by Gallaudet University Press in an abbreviated picture book format with line drawings.

Her delight was evident when the librarian signed *Jack and the Beanstalk* (Galdone). Then, using the flannel board, the librarian related *The Monkey and the Crocodile* (Galdone), during which the child signed for both animals. At story's end, she clapped and laughed. For fifteen minutes, she had enjoyed communicative company and an intermission in her isolation.

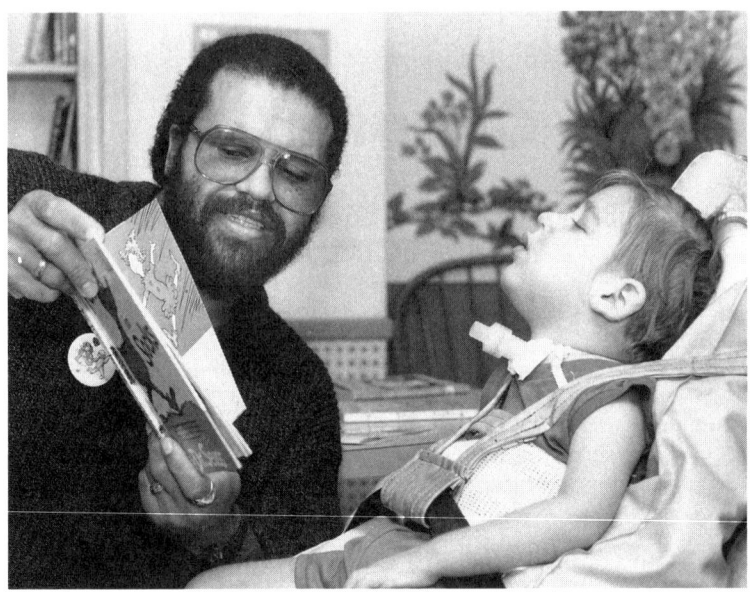

A child life specialist reads aloud to a child with special needs.

Michael — A Child with Vision Impairment

Learning that the child read Braille, the librarian carried a stack of picture books in Braille to the doorway of eight-year-old Michael's room. "Who is there?" he asked. In this situation, it is especially important to identify yourself promptly. Michael and his mother were pleased to have Braille books to read in the hospital.

A visually impaired child not yet strong in Braille skills is a good candidate for a read-aloud time. Select stories involving the senses of smell, taste, touch, and sound, like *The Very Quiet Cricket* (Carle) and *The Very Busy Spider* (Carle). Stories about successes large and small are also recommended. Books on tape are generally available from stores and the public library.

Mahogany — A Child with Quadriplegia

The first time the librarian saw this four-year-old child, who was critically injured in a car accident, she awakened only occasionally during a reading of *Whistle for Willie* (Keats). When the librarian used the flannel board to tell *The Man Who Did Not Wash His Dishes* (Krasilovsky), the child's nurse rubbed her cheeks and the librarian spoke more loudly. After she stayed awake for the entire story, her nurse and the librarian clapped for her. Her response was a wide smile.

On the second visit, large tears ran down the child's cheeks as the librarian read *Ask Mr. Bear* (Flack). Did she miss her mother? The child life specialist assured the librarian it was all right that Mahogany cried — she needed to cry. A safe space with the librarian is a good place to air feelings.

On the third visit, she laughed at *Dear Zoo* (Campbell) and took pleasure in finding the cat in *Angus and the Cat* (Flack). She was more animated and responsive, said her child life specialist, than she had been for days.

The day before the child's transfer to a rehabilitation center, the librarian gave a puppet show of *The Gingerbread Boy* (Galdone). The medical staff and others had been trying to encourage her to turn her head. When the gingerbread boy ran across the kitchen floor and out the door, the child moved her head. During one of the chases, she did it again.

Emma — A Child with a Head Injury

A truck hit an Amish buggy, sending a family of seven flying through the air. One child, age nine, landed on a roadside mailbox and sustained a severe head injury. It was questionable whether she could see or hear.

When the librarian entered the room, she lay motionless. Then she was placed in a wheelchair and held upright by straps.

The librarian began reading *The Big Red Barn* (Brown). Did she see the kitten on the page? Slowly, her eyes followed the librarian's finger down to a lower corner of the colorful illustration.

Elated, the librarian read on, choosing *The Josefina Story Quilt* (Coerr), another familiar object with which an Amish child could make a connection.

Emma continued to listen intently, occasionally flipping her braid. She looked directly at the librarian when the read-aloud time had ended.

A few days later, Emma was tranferred to another hospital to be near her mother. A follow-up phone call to the director of child life there encouraged continued reading aloud.

Carlos and Haynes — Young People with Developmental Delay

Four-year-old Carlos moved restlessly in his cart. When the librarian started reading *The Tale of Peter Rabbit* (Potter), he was as still as Peter himself watching from the wheelbarrow. Whenever the librarian paused between books, he whimpered for more.

A year later, he returned to the hospital. His mother was gratified that the librarian knew Carlos and showed an interest in him. Readily, she accepted a nursery rhyme book to read aloud, perhaps happy that she had been shown a way to interact with her child.

Twenty-two-year-old Haynes came to Story Hour wearing a baseball T-shirt and a large diaper. He threw back his head and laughed appropriately at funny parts in the story. Later in his room, his foster mother asked for picture books for him. *Could Anything Be Worse?* (Hirsh) and *Lazy Jack* (Ross) seemed good choices because the main characters are adults. Remembering his sense of humor, the librarian encouraged his mother to try *Mr. Popper's Penguins* (Atwater). Later that day, she met the mother on the stairway. "Chapter books!" the mother exclaimed. "I never knew he could follow them."

A librarian telling stories during Story Hour is soon aware of nonverbal patients who are developmentally delayed. Sometimes, these children will become animated and murmur along with the story telling. A wide smile on seeing the librarian again reminds one that, while these children may not have expressive speech, they seem to have receptive understanding, and Story Hour can be a source of real pleasure for them.

When reading to a child who is developmentally delayed, the following suggestions may be helpful:

Choose books with a strong story line — straightforward action and an evident beginning, middle, and end. If necessary, shorten the story, but keep the plot intact.

Substitute the child's name for the name of the main character; this helps to make a connection.

Read slowly and with expression. Don't hurry — this listener especially needs time to process and create mental pictures.

Jason — A Child in a Comatose State

It requires belief in what one is doing to take a book into the room of a comatose patient. Usually the light is dim, sometimes the radio is on, the room is usually empty of parents and visitors.

The patient seldom moves. Does he hear anything? A volunteer reader told the librarian: "I acted toward Jason as though he were a normal child and he sighed when Peter finally learned to whistle." In reading to the comatose child, it is important to keep these things in mind.

Medical specialists cannot be absolutely certain of a definitive prognosis following a serious brain injury, but it is certain that "the speed and success of intervention often affect the eventual outcome."[1] It is known also that the young brain's "flexibility, teamed with a drive to succeed and the help of a supportive environment can generate seemingly miraculous results."[2]

Patients are still able to hear when they have lost other faculties; thus reading aloud to the child may provide specific benefits. Talking about the pictures to the child may encourage responses to the described images.

Reading to the comatose child probably reaches him on a cerebral level that is different from the level responding to loud repetitions of "Wake up! Jason. Can you hear me?"

For the parent fatigued from anxiety, frustration, and one-way conversations, reading aloud brings relaxation, pleasure, and a needed sense of doing something to help that is an appropriate activity between parent and child.

If, during the reading aloud, the reader notices any changes in response, notify the staff so that the response is noted on the patient's chart.

Don't be afraid of physical contact. Gently rub the child's arm or tap his hand. Be careful not to disturb an IV.

Prepare carefully! Choose a book from a fairly low reading level, particularly a story he may remember. Work hard to make connections of any kind. Read from an author his family says he especially likes. If he had a particular interest in any subject just prior to his hospitalization, choose a book from that subject area. In this situation too, replace the main character's name with the child's name.

April — A Young Adolescent with Neurological Devastation

A teenage girl showed no responses after suffering a virulent infection. Following six weeks on a ventilator in the intensive care unit with a DNR (Do Not Resuscitate) order, she was diagnosed as neurologically devastated.

Her mother encouraged the child life specialist to read to April. During the reading of *Superfudge* (Blume), she blinked her eyes. When asked to close her eyes, she did so. In response to the question, "Do you like books?" she nodded slightly.

"Do you like Judy Blume?"

"Uh-huh."

"I think she's coming out of it," her mother exclaimed.

The child life specialist's notes in the patient's chart led the neurologist to tell his interns in the hall, "We know now to be careful what we say in that room."

Crystal — A Child with a Terminal Illness

The extent to which the librarian becomes involved with a child who is dying depends largely on her relationship with the child and parents. In order to work effectively with a dying child, one must be keenly aware of one's own emotional limitations. One may be already overwhelmed with personal problems or painful memories. It is wise to judge one's readiness for involvement.

A five-year-old child was diagnosed with cancer. Uncared for by her parents, she was placed in a foster home.

In the six months she lived with her loving foster family, her extended hospitalizations increased. During this period, she still went regularly to Story Hour. It was only when she worsened significantly that she could no longer be brought to the library.

When the librarian took books to her, she wanted only familiar titles. Perhaps it took less effort to follow stories she already knew. Perhaps there was some reassurance in them. After each visit, she gave the librarian a sticker or a drawing. Maybe during her last days, she was learning about giving and receiving kindness. Perhaps, also, she simply wanted to insure the librarian's return.

The librarian shared the Story Hour activities. Once, though greatly weakened, Crystal leaned forward from her pillow to make the effort — a happy, willing effort — to plant beans in a soil-filled cup. Her eyes followed the librarian as she placed the cup on the window sill.

When death was imminent, she no longer wanted the librarian to read to her. Occasionally, she reached out to stroke the Story Hour puppet's head. The librarian's presence seemed to be all she wanted.

Chang and Nicholas — Children with Ventilator Dependency

Chang, a very young child with ventilator dependency, has been hospitalized for the first two years of his life. Dependent on a ventilator, he lacks mobility and misses out on normal situations encountered by other children.

Because this child cannot come to Toddler/Preschool Story Hour at an appropriate age, it is important to take Story Hour to him. The child should be given the chance to remove and replace flannel board figures and to interact with lift-and-see books. Puppets elicit a special response. Finger/hand play is important to help encourage motor skills. Exposure to nursery rhymes and to stories with rhyme and repetition is helpful. "A child who has absorbed...the melody of language is statistically destined to have an easier time learning to read."[3]

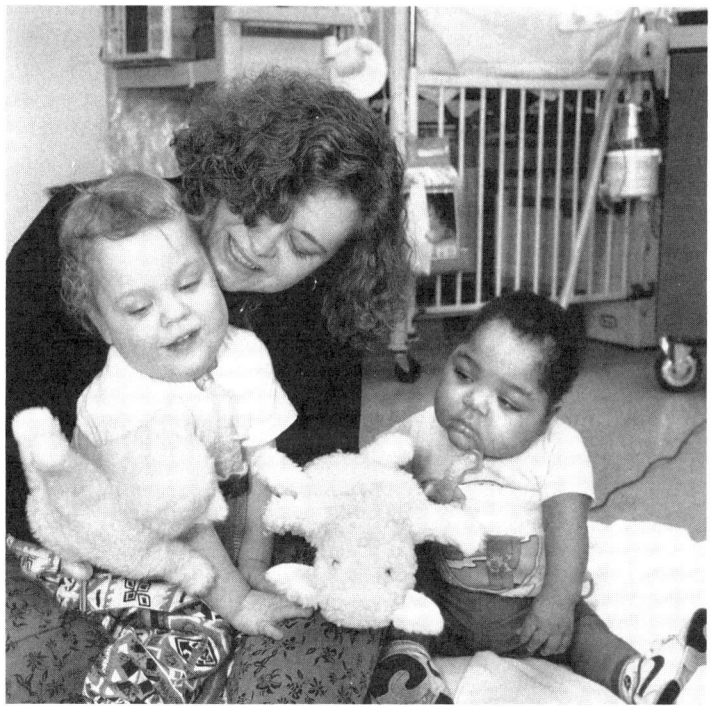

Ventilator-dependent children and a child life specialist play with puppets.

Like his peers, Chang can learn about simple objects, colors, and the five senses, but his experiences are very limited. The child life specialist and librarian can cooperate in bringing in objects that match the illustrations in books like: *Of Colors and Things* (Hoban).

Nicholas, a six-year-old child with bronchopulmonary dysplasia at home again following yet another hospital stay, asked his mother as she tucked him into bed, "Who will be my night nurse?" — a telling question from a "hospital child" — revealing his lack of family consistency amd consequent confusion related to hospitalization. *Blueberries for Sal* (McCloskey) and *The Stories Julian Tells* (Cameron) are recommended family stories for reading aloud to this child.

Helping to meet the unique developmental needs of the ventilator dependent child is a special challenge for the librarian and other staff. "…those who work with children must insure that there is an enriched environment in order for individual children to grow and mature."[4] One does not know what goes through a child's mind. What a librarian can know is that the child benefits from her consistent visits and from her use of quality materials — touchstones of the librarians's work with any child — but especially so with the hospitalized child with special needs.

Chapter 9.

THE BOOK CART
ON THE PATIENT FLOORS

When the librarian or volunteer steps off the elevator into a maze of children, families, and staff members, she is immediately identified by the book cart.

ASPECTS OF THE BOOK CART SERVICE

The book cart should be large enough to hold an assortment of materials, yet low and small enough for young patients to reach the books without assistance. Each end of the cart can display an identifying sign like "Kids' Library," indicating also the library's hours and location. Stocking one side of the cart with books for the young child and the other side with materials for the older patient seems to work well. Mylar balloons to celebrate events like "Children's Book Week" and colorful posters tell the patient that this is not an EKG monitor coming through the door. Wearing a special apron, button pin, or hat can also identify the librarian or "book person."

It can be hard not to feel intimidated by busy, preoccupied members of the medical staff, but most staff members recognize the value of the psychosocial service provided by the librarian and the book cart.

Sometimes on seeing the book cart, a child will smile for the first time that day or leap up from a prone position and dash over to the cart. Other patients will be too medicated or ill to respond. Sometimes talking with the child's parent, visitor, or nurse will help the librarian to choose books to leave on the bedside table for the time the child is feeling better. Inquiries at the nurses' station help to direct the librarian selecting books for patients in isolation. Teen and children's magazines that can be tossed out are good choices for the patient in contagion.

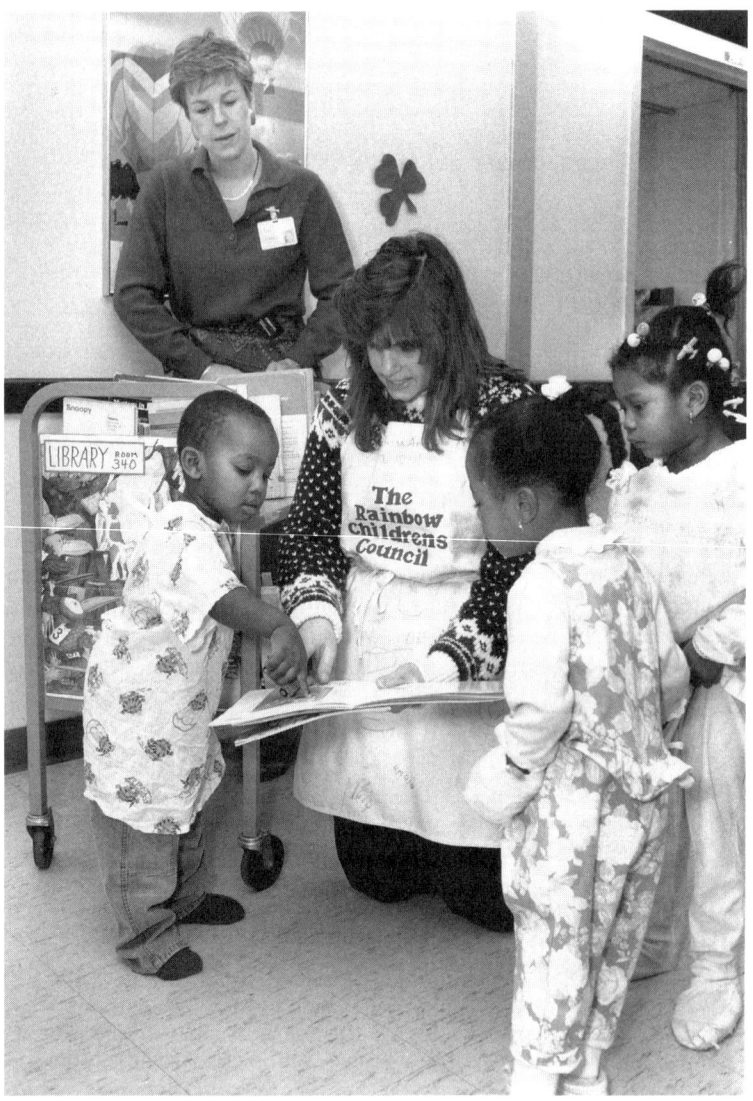

A child who is out of his room for treatment is happy to return to find books on his bed or may look forward to returning to them. Other children can take the books along with them to medical tests and the long waiting times.

Occasionally a child will reject the book cart. Perhaps it is the first thing all day he's been able to say "no" to. Respect his need to feel that, at least in this instance, he is in charge. A more common experience is the patient who is simply not feeling up to making decisions. A few gentle questions and showing of books help this child to make appropriate choices.

Stop your rounds to read to any child who is crying and alone. Some children will ask you to read to them.

Sometimes the librarian discerns a patient's interests by noting what the child is drawing. A nine-year-old playing with astronaut figures in the playroom led to lending him books on space. This is not to say that a number of patients do not know exactly what they want. Once the librarian approached the bedside of a motorcycle casualty who announced loudly: "I like street books. See?"

The book cart is an entrée to talking with parents and to being a good listener. Sometimes your presence triggers a question regarding their child's homework assignment and requests for supplemental materials. Other times this is the chance to talk about the Family Resource Collection.

Try to make a good match between parent and child when suggesting a book. Sometimes, this is a first opportunity for a parent to read aloud to her child; it could be the start of a fruitful habit.

Be ready to offer "call backs" — a return to the child with specially requested materials. The child should be assured that if the librarian does not return, it is because the books are not available — he was not forgotten. Prepare him also for the fact that "call backs" take place later in the day.

Hand out book lists, bookmarks, and quizzes or puzzles relating to books. This helps promote reading. (See Resources.)

NOT ALWAYS EASY

It can honestly be said that going onto the patient floors is not always easy. What is easy is staying in the library — but that is not the place for the librarian in a pediatric setting. Like the child life specialist, the librarian does not distance herself from the patients. She is responsive to and involved in meeting their needs. Until you devise your own coping skills, some of the following procedural suggestions will be helpful.

If the patient is receiving medical care, do not interrupt; make a note to return after finishing your rounds on the rest of the floor. The same holds true if the child and family are giving a medical history or if the patient is being examined.

In particular, adolescent and adult patients value their privacy. Even if the door is open, knock before entering. All patients grow tired of intrusions but are usually pleased to see the librarian.

Sometimes one will enter a room to see a patient who is in very bad shape. A good practice is to return to the hallway to collect one's thoughts on what to say to the patient or his family. Often, approaching a roommate who is in better condition gives you a chance to assess the situation in the next bed. Perhaps the family would be better served than the patient. Perhaps it is better not to return to the room — a talk with the nurse may provide the information that a child is in crisis.

Most difficult situations are balanced by positive experiences: families eager to see the librarian again, patients happy to learn about the library for the first time, young people with varying disabilities who are candidates for special materials that are available, the chance to talk about the zoo animals coming to Story Hour.

Children like books. When approached, they are quickly aware that the librarian is a friend, not a threat. Knowing this helps both patient and librarian to make an easy relationship that speaks to the patient's interests and affirms his normalcy. Follow cues given by the child's reaction on seeing the book cart, sometimes tactfully ignoring a parent's hesitation or lack of interest.

In spite of difficult moments, going onto the floors can be a high point of the librarian's work. The book cart service is a non-threatening interlude in the day and a time of human contact. Like many opportunities provided by the child life program and other therapies, the book cart service gives young patients a chance to be children through books and juvenile magazines, and gives adolescent patients a chance to be teenagers again.

Chapter 10.

BIBLIOTHERAPY WITH HOSPITALIZED CHILDREN

"Bibliotherapy is a way to help children cope with life,"[1] states Doris Robinson, a children's librarian, who is a member of the American Library Association's (ALA) Bibliotherapy Forum. In l988, the Association of Specialized and Co-operative Library Agencies (ASCLA), a division of ALA, accepted the following definition of bibliotherapy: "...a discussion process guided by a facilitator using literature as the catalyst to promote insight, normal development, and rehabilitation."

In a hospital setting, the person interacting between the child and the book can be a child life specialist, nurse, or a volunteer reader who is supervised by the librarian. In this setting, bibliotherapy is practiced with children who are experiencing a medical trauma, personal crisis, or more common life problem, such as moving to a new home.

Because many children's hospital stays are brief, full follow-up discussion is rarely possible; but often, by identifying with a character and situation, the child may learn a coping skill, an attitude change, or insight into a problem's resolution. Hospitalized children should have access to books that offer these possibilities.

Noted bibliotherapist Margaret Hannigan has cautioned that bibliotherapy "is therapeutic rather than therapy."[2] "Bibliotherapy exists as a tool within the many spheres of therapy."[3]

One of the intrinsic strengths of literature is that it cannot be twisted for specific uses. The reader will take from it only what reaches him, what touches his sensibilities and understanding. No matter what its use, the book survives as a story first, as something written from the heart, as one person's vision, as an imagined world with identifiable characters. A child's inner life can relate to a book and be nourished. "Books relating to a child's inner needs combined with story experiences initiated by thoughtful, caring adults, can and frequently do help children grow."[4]

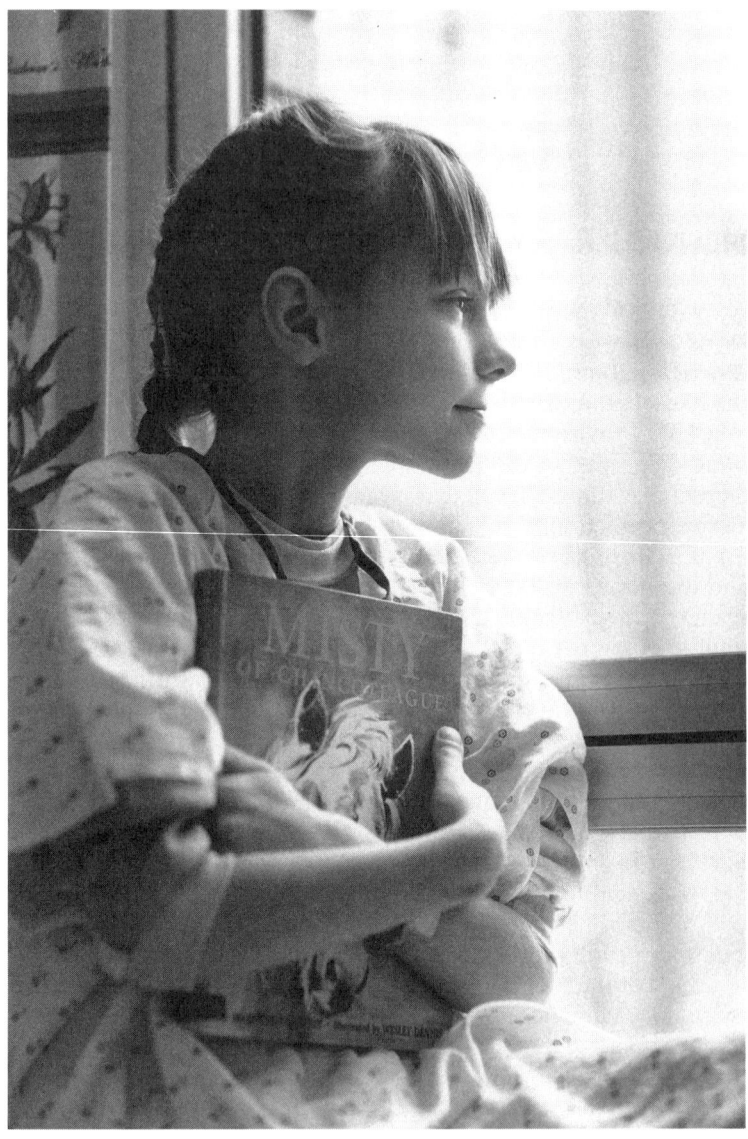

Book depicted: *Misty of Chincoteague*, by Marguerite Henry, illustrated by Wesley
Dennis. New York: Macmillan Publishing Company, 1947, 1975. Used with permission
of the publisher.

ADDRESSING COMMON EMOTIONS THROUGH FICTION

Books and stories speak to children in many different ways. Children know what they want to read and when they want to read it. For this reason, public and hospital libraries now organize special concerns shelves where young readers can make their own choices. Following their instincts, children have a more accurate sense of timing and of topic than has the most well-meaning adult.

Author Katherine Paterson has written of every child's "inarticulate fears."[5] The hospitalized child experiences heightened unexpressed hopes, instincts for survival, feelings of loneliness, sadness, and loss. "Make-believe is the key that helps a child unlock his feelings."[6]

Robinson reminds us that it is better to read about life's traumas before they happen. A librarian does not usually read of death and dying to a child in the "end stage" of a chronic illness. A year before she died of cystic fibrosis, a child asked specifically for *Charlotte's Web* (White). Did she know something about the story, she was asked. Yes, she said. She did. Perhaps this child was following her own accurate instincts.

It is also better to read a book that speaks to the emotion rather than one that mirrors the specific trauma. A ten-year-old child seriously injured in a car accident appeared to be inordinately fearful, even though her recovery was going smoothly. Through further inquiry, it was learned that her grandmother had died recently in a hospital. Rather than address the trauma by reading a book like *Saying Goodbye to Gramma* (Thomas), the reader chose a book about feeling fearful: *Storm in the Night* (Stolz). A book like this can reach a child on two levels: one, that she is not alone in feeling fearful; and two, that many of the things we fear never happen.

Using picture books is especially recommended. The illustrations can evoke emotions that words do not.

Sometimes, exposure to books in general can reassure a child and lead to stress reduction — a component of wellness and recovery. For example, Isaac, a five-year-old, was badly injured in a traffic accident and traumatized to the extent that he opposed physically and hysterically all medical interventions on his behalf. After three days, he still shrieked at the sight of medical personnel. His response was of special concern to his primary care nurses. The more frightened the child became, the more his parents surrounded him with the strictures of their orthodox religious faith. Medical staff, child life, and the hospital chaplain had all tried vainly to establish a therapeutic relationship with the child.

As a last resort, the librarian was asked to take in some books for Isaac because he had expressed an interest in Story Hour. Anticipating his screams and somewhat unnerved by all the warnings regarding him, she held open picture books as she entered his room, so there would be no doubt as to her role in the hospital.

He was whimpering when she approached his bed. With a strong grasp, he pulled the books from her hold before she finished her introduction. "And would you like to see the filmstrip of *The Little House* (Burton) we saw in Story Hour?" she asked then. He would.

During the quiet conversation with him and his mother, Isaac's primary care nurse approached the bed. Without incident, she rearranged Isaac's pillows and smiled at him.

A few minutes later, a nurse, not believing the quiet from Isaac's room, said to the librarian, "You haven't gone in yet, have you?"

From this initial contact and other variables, the child opened gradually to a more trusting relationship with other staff members. Isaac knew books; they were his friends. If there were books around, the hospital could not be such a terrible place after all. Perhaps, he may have deduced, there were even people in the hospital who could help him.

ADDRESSING COMMON EMOTIONS THROUGH INFORMATIONAL NONFICTION AND DIDACTIC FICTION

In recent years, much informational nonfiction and didactic fiction has been published addressing children's emotions. In this literature, the concern is addressed directly in a way that can add to a child's stress. As stated earlier, children will make the right selection with these books too.

One of the major values of this literature is providing the words needed by the child to express feelings. The right words can be helpful to parents too.

ADDRESSING DEVELOPMENTAL GROWTH

For the long-term hospitalized child, bibliotherapy can have a definite educational orientation. Developmental bibliotherapy is a fairly common practice in pediatric settings. Sometimes, parents concentrate all their energies on their child's illness and fail to prepare their child for ordinary life transitions: entry into school,

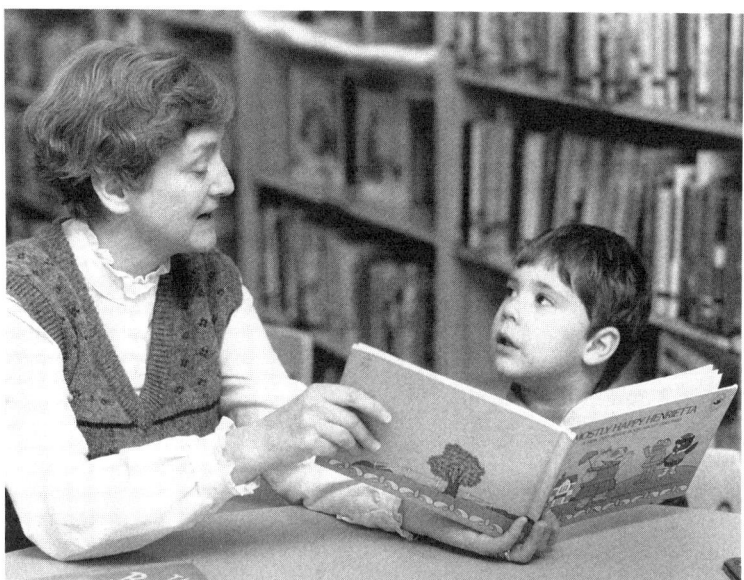

a new home, etc. Identifying with book characters coping with these transitions helps the reader to experience them too. Bibliotherapy proves its specific help to the long-term patient — a "hospital child" — one whose lengthy confinement has robbed him of many months of cognitive development, everyday life experiences, personal relationships with people other than fellow patients and medical staff, and knowledge of the natural world.

Adam was admitted so that serious surgery could be performed to prolong his life, threatened by a rare disease. Consequently, he spent thirteen consecutive months in our hospital; previous to this surgery, he had experienced several long-term hospitalizations in another hospital.

During his long recovery, he started first grade in the hospital school. Learning to read was difficult for him. In an effort to support the struggle to acquire a skill crucial for a child with a limited capacity for activity and to keep alive his obvious enjoyment of books, Adam started coming into the library twice a week for what he called his "library time."

The first two times he came, his experiential deprivations were apparent, particularly in three specific areas: experiences with seasons and holidays outside the hospital walls (he remembered no

Christmas at home); the natural environment: weather, plants, and animals; and normal family relationships.

He began with stories about holidays and the four seasons. Perhaps because holidays are often made much of in pediatric settings, he looked forward to them many weeks in advance. Halloween and Christmas were anchor lines in the twilight hours of medications, the unreal environment of intensive care, and a dimly lit hospital room. Yet, holidays in the hospital are not like holidays at home. Through books like: *Seasons* (Goennel) and *When Summer Ends* (Fowler), Adam was exposed to around-the-year seasons and celebrations.

To help him and other children stay in touch with the natural environment, the librarian used more nature in Story Hour and shelf decor. Planted seeds, daffodils, sea shells, fossils, and interesting stones were used in Story Hour activities as Take-Aways and as library displays. *What Will the Weather Be Like Today?* (Rogers) and *Keep Looking* (Selsam) were books of particular interest.

Certain books addressed Adam's lack of familiarity with animals. This was a significant handicap in his early efforts to read, for many beginning readers feature animals as main characters. He did not know a domestic animal from a wild animal; he had never been to a farm or a zoo. It was not surprising that early reading materials elicited little response.

After many readings, some of his best-loved books were Lobel's *Frog and Toad* series. Aside from being amusing, these animals were dependable; he trusted them. When a live frog appeared at Story Hour, he was not disillusioned. The last day he came to his "library time," he was asked what special words he wanted written for him to post on his bedside wall. He replied: "Frog said, 'Get well, Adam.' "

The third and most serious void in his experience was his minimal knowledge of a loving, caring family. His mother's excuse for not visiting was that she was too busy working — a common enough reason given during the work week. Adam's father and brother came rarely. No one came on his birthday. Adam's most beloved story was *Noisy Nora* (Wells). Ignored by a preoccupied family and a mother who is busy with a new baby, Nora tries to attract attention to herself by becoming a noisy nuisance. Failing at that, she "leaves home" and disappears into a broom closet. Her family searches frantically for her and great is their joy at her sudden reappearance. Perhaps, Adam identified primarily with Nora's feelings of rejection. "Nora is really mad, isn't she?" he said, pointing to a picture of Nora knocking down a floor lamp. "If I were her mother, I'd work faster. Then I'd have the time to give Nora."

Charlotte Zolotow's sensitive books, *If It Weren't for You*, *Big Brother*, and *Do You Know What I'll Do?* were especially effective introductions to sibling feelings and interactions.

Armed with a personal copy of *Noisy Nora*, Adam returned to his home in July. By summer's end, he was placed with a foster family, where over time he began to feel comfortable.

In late November, Adam walked again into Story Hour. Sitting quietly in a chair, he smiled and said simply, "I want some books."

Adam borrowed *Corduroy* (Freeman), a book he had heard several times in Story Hour. Perhaps now, he understood the feelings of a lonely, stuffed bear bought from a department store by a little girl. " 'This must be a home,' said Corduroy [carried tightly in the little girl's arms to her bedroom]. 'I know I've always wanted a home.' "

GUIDELINES FOR WORKING WITH CHILDREN THROUGH BOOKS

Affirm the child with whom you are working. Reassure the child that anything she talks about is private.

Let the conversation occur easily. Do not press for a response. "Listening with empathy offers children maximum opportunity for expression."[7]

Make it clear that all her thoughts and questions are important, natural, and occur to other children too — and that she is respected for them.

Listen and respond to questions. If the child does not ask questions, ask open-ended questions yourself. In all cases, give an honest answer even if it is: "I don't know."

At times, validating feelings helps to cement a relationship between you and the child.

Further guidelines and support materials can be found in the Resources section. Bibliotherapy titles are available at many public libraries.

Chapter 11.

POETRY WRITING IN A PEDIATRIC SETTING

Hospitalized children express themselves in many ways through their art, play, music, and writings. Of their varied writings, poetry offers the most immediate impact for the reader and listener because of its brevity, emotional overtones, and pointedness.[1]

The rationale for encouraging writing poetry is that it provides for catharsis — a relieving of emotional tensions — which is generally beneficial to the hospitalized child and young adult.

A scheduled poetry writing time within the library program offers young patients an opportunity for self-expression and a chance to enhance self-esteem. Patients come for reasons of their own: writing a poem sounds like fun; a teacher might give extra credit; writing poetry is a favorite pastime; the afternoon is lonely on the floor...

Writing poetry can also be an escape from the limitations of illness and disability and a break from medical protocol. That poetry writing can be pleasurable was shown by a young asthmatic who said, "I was having so much fun, I forgot to use my oxygen."

The accomplishment of a poem affords a child the opportunity to be a "poet" rather than a "diabetic" or a "paraplegic." Respect and interest are usually prompt responses from fellow patients and adults.

ORIGINAL POETRY

An eleven-year-old boy with a history of sleep disturbances and school absenteeism wrote the following poem:

A trip to Mars, a trip to Mars.
There wouldn't be any trucks or cars.
A trip to Mars would have strange beings,
No one there to hurt your feelings.

There would be nothing out there to weigh you down,
There would be no cities or fancy towns.
Out there you could see many stars.
Boy, what a great trip to Mars.

The child escaped through this poem by way of an imagined journey.
Later, with the help of counseling, he learned to cope with some
hard realities in his life.

An anorexic on her way to "recovery" described what she saw
in her mirror. Her poem supported studies that indicate that rail
thin anorexic/bulimic patients actually see themselves as "fat."

Mirror, why did you stare at me
and announce all my flaws? Your placid face
bellowed out every insecurity until I hated me.

I cried because you knew how easily I
broke. You laughed and screamed, "Indulgence,
lazy, corpulence" — as the light reflected
from every rib and bone.

Then, I saw a baby before a mirror.
Smiling, he crawled to his reflection and
kissed it. "Baby," he proudly explained.

Mirror, your face has smudged. I see
you now as only glass.

A group or collaborative poem was written by four adolescent
boys, ages thirteen to fifteen. They were an angry group and the
poetry leader was an easy target for their hostility. In a hard situation like this, one can only continue, and cling to the possibilities
of the finished poem. Gradually, finding an absence of hostile
response from the poetry leader, the focus changed, the content
shifted. When the writing time was over, they turned their
wheelchairs without a word and left the library.

After the poem was typed, the poets received copies. Each
poet was subdued and pleased. "You mean," said one smiling, "our
poem is on the Poetry Door?"

I wish for a better place to live —
cleaner streets

no writing on the walls
quieter trucks
I wish for money and a red van
I wish I could beat up my older brother
and blow up my principal's car
I wish for no more headaches
I wish for peace
I wish for a falling star.

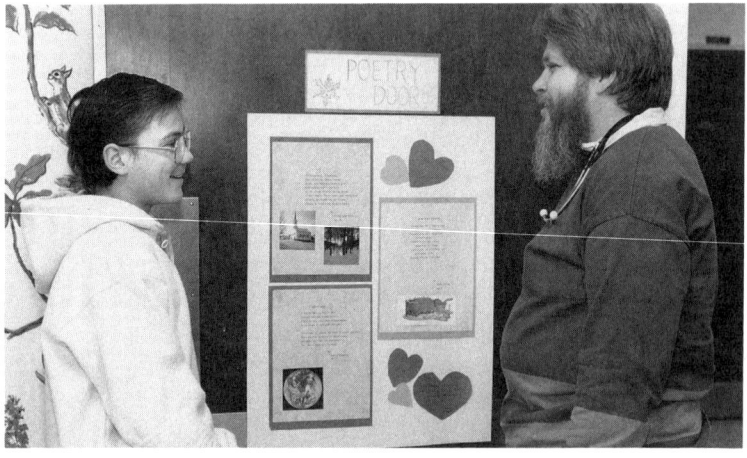

A patient and nurse enjoy the poetry door.

The following poem expresses an adolescent's sadness at isolation from activities and separation from family and friends. In the last verse, the poet expresses hope by concretizing in her own words what she has been told by the medical staff.

I've been here a while
And I can hardly keep my smile.
It's gradually getting harder and harder.

They say every day, "You're doing so well."
But I'm getting discouraged and don't feel
all that swell,
I just want to get better.

Last summer I had such a great time,
But this summer isn't as sublime.
I'd like to go home.

But I realize I have to stay here a bit longer
So next summer I will feel a lot stronger,
And I can have a good time once again.

Four children ages seven through eleven wrote the following
group poem about the hospital experience. Sometimes, a poem like
this provides an opportunity to address misconceptions about the
hospital.

In my imagined hospital day...
I would break all the needles and throw
    them away.
I would hide the doctors' white coats
    and ID cards
And sprinkle the doctors with magic powder
    to make them midgets.
Then the kids would be the docs and
    they'd know how we feel!
In my imagined hospital day...
I would make Becky, the two-month-old
    baby in my room get well.
I would eat pancakes and french toast
    for breakfast.
I would make a model of the hospital
    with tongue depressors, climb to the
    top of it, and fly away...
In my imagined hospital day.

Line by line, this next poet expresses a mixture of feelings commonly experienced by hospitalized children: anger, altruism,
idealism, and empathy.

If I were a lion, I would bite
    somebody's head off.
If I were a doctor, I would take
    care of all my patients.
If I were a star, I would be a
    bright star.
If I were a door, I would not like
    to be slammed shut.

W   inter

I   s very

N   ear, so near

T   hat I can almost see

E   very snowflake and hear the

R   eindeer on my roof.

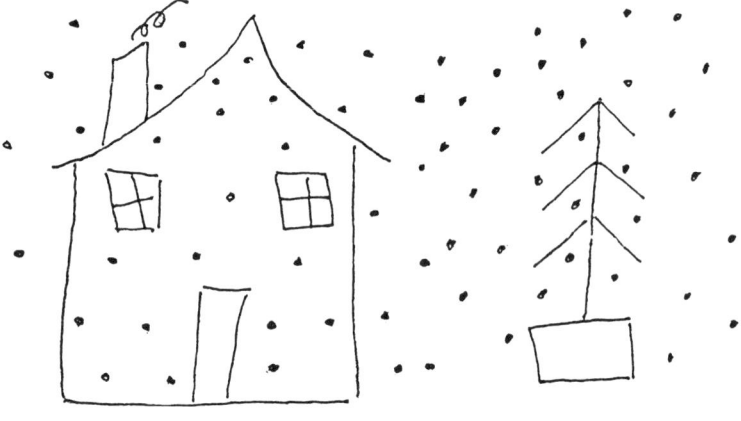

A page from the poetry anthology written and illustrated by young patients.

The last poem was written by a teenage cystic fibrosis patient shortly before she died. She told her child life specialist that she longed to see snow one more time. Like other patients in the end stage of their illnesses, the poet turned to nature — and found in snow a metaphor for death and dying.

> Out the window, in the dusk,
> Snow is falling, quiet, hushed.
> Bright moon shining with white glow,
> Highlighting soft drifts below.
> Drifts piling, blowing, moving around,
> As more fragile flakes drift down, down, down,
> Covering the fields and the streams,
> Leaving my world a sea of white dreams.

METHODS FOR ENCOURAGING WRITING

Ideas flow more easily if the writing is done in a non-threatening environment, such as the library. In any setting, mutual trust must be established in a short time. It is essential that the poet experience a sense of personal support and encouragement in the process of expressing himself. The poetry leader should write also, thus sharing in the vulnerability.

Grammar and spelling should not be major concerns. Some patients will need help with their handwriting; a few, especially younger children, may dictate. In an effort to support self-assertion, one poetry leader said, "You be the boss and I'll write it down."

Reading aloud a few poems written by other young patients or by professional poets can lead to subject ideas.

An assortment of pictures or artifacts can awaken sensibilities and memories and thus encourage creativity.

Some sessions might begin with writing a group poem. Subject discussion leads to a choice of topic statements, such as: "I secretly like...," "When I'm in the hospital...," and "Where I would rather be...."

Rhyme is not important, but many poets like to rhyme at least the first or last few lines. "It seems more like a poem now" is a frequent comment.

Poetry can be meaningful and effective in a single sentence. A young patient in New York's Bellevue Hospital wrote: "Sadness comes in the night like an owl."

Younger poets, ages 8 to 12, like to write "shape poems," where the words follow a simple figure like a baseball bat or an IV pole. Haiku is also a popular poetic form.

Young adult and adult poets will often choose free verse to encourage the flow and feeling of freedom needed to address difficult personal issues and concerns.

Encouraging the use of specific details, e.g., color, size, and all the five senses helps to create imagery.

AFTER WRITING

The poet is encouraged to read the poem aloud. Be supportive of the poem. Ask to hear it read twice. Poems are meant to be read aloud. Suggestions for changes are made only after a sensitive assessment of both the poet and the poem, and should be presented simply as a means of improving clarity and avoiding cliches.

If the poetry leader encourages poets to add a few personal feelings, many are willing to do so — provided the atmosphere is deemed a safe one. A promise of confidentiality is sometimes a prerequisite; but more often than not, poets are open about their feelings.

All poems are typed for distribution and for posting on the Poetry Door. Very rarely does a poet choose anonymity or refuse presentation of her work. Record the poets' names, addresses, and ages before concluding poetry writing time. In our hospital, a representative collection of the children's writing and illustrations is published every two years.

USES OF ORIGINAL POETRY

That a poem has been written at all is reason enough for its existence! If, however, there is interest in publishing a collection of selected poems or in using the poems as part of a hospital's public relations program, the following steps should be taken.

Solicit legal help to formulate a release form to be signed by parents or adult patients giving permission to use original poetry in a variety of ways.

If, due to many reasons, release forms do not get signed, print a disclaimer in any publication containing the poems. A sample appears below:

> This book is published solely
> for distribution for educational
> purposes and is not intended for
> sale to the general public.

Enlist assistance early from the hospital's development or public relations office. Sources of funding may be varied, but can include: a state arts council; family or community foundations; a literary non-profit organization such as Poets in Public Service; private contributions. The Rockefeller Center subway station in New York City provided space for a multipanel display of poetry and art by young patients at St. Mary's Hospital for Children, Queens, NY.

A FEW ASSESSMENTS

The poetry writing program appears to mean much to young patients. Follow up is seen in a number of unsolicited letters. One poet expressed her thanks for "easing the initial fears of a hospital stay by offering time to write poetry and explore emotions through literature."

Another wrote: "Although my eating behavior sometimes gets out of hand every once in a while, I have found solace, comfort, and even control through creative writing."

However young patients are exposed to poetry — that written by others and their own — they learn that people share common feelings and gain a sense of mastery by putting their emotions into written words. Together, they take part in a subconscious pursuit of what has been called in children's poetry "a search for wholeness."[2]

FURTHER ASSISTS

Consult the Resources section for helpful guides to writing poetry.

A number of poetry collections are named in Chapter 6. Below are a few other recommended titles:

'Til All the Stars Have Fallen (Booth)
A Week in the Life of Best Friends (de Regniers)
The Road Not Taken (Frost)
Class Dismissed!: High School Poems (Glenn)
Honey, I Love and other Love Poems and Nathanial Talking
   (Greenfield)

Poems for Small Friends (Katz)
Where the Sidewalk Ends plus other titles (Silverstein)
Street Talk (Turner)
All the Small Poems (Worth)

Nurses

Nurses are patient,
Nurses are kind,
Nurses help you to relax
And to ease your mind.

They help you out
When times are rough.
They stick by you
when the going gets tough.

So if you ever need one
To care and share,
Just remember a nurse.
She'll always be there.

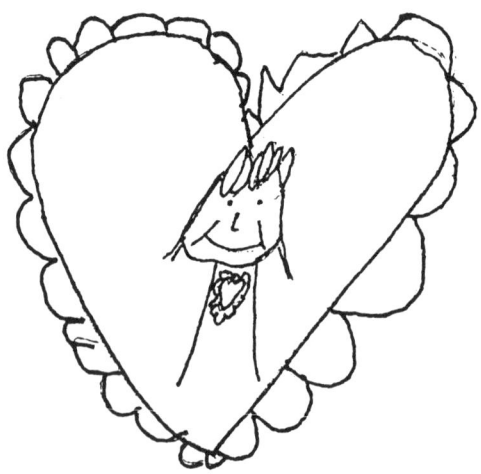

Poem and illustration by young patients.

Chapter 12.

A FAMILY RESOURCE COLLECTION

A Family Resource Collection is based on the premise that family centered care is a desirable goal and that knowledgeable parents are resourceful and supportive partners in the multidisciplinary care of their child.

"Most families, when faced with a crisis, go through a series of responses to the problem in a consistent pattern." During this "process of adaptation," families usually reach a "focusing outward" stage: "a time of energy renewal when family members seek information and options for the child's future."[1] At this point, the Family Resource Collection is of special value.

The general purposes of a Family Resource Collection are:

1. To supplement information provided by the health care staff.
2. To help families develop coping skills with respect to the diagnosis of their child's illness or disability.
3. To encourage and support the family in participating in the treatment process.

Besides using the Collection to obtain information, parents and sometimes siblings have opportunities to air their anxieties and to clear up misunderstandings. In both instances, the librarian can encourage the family to talk again with the health care staff, where the primary nurse should be a coordinator of the concerns raised by the family. A child life specialist and a social worker should be on call for further consultation and counseling, if necessary.

Sometimes, a parent understands the child's situation better when given the opportunity to quietly read selected and appropriate materials.

GUIDELINES AND BIBLIOGRAPHIES

Guidelines for Establishing a Family Resource Library —

Second Edition is published by the Association for the Care of Children's Health (ACCH). This invaluable resource is a highly recommended purchase providing — among other topics — information on planning, funding, space, policies and procedures, acquisition and processing, outreach and promotion. *Reference to this text will be your best guide in establishing a Family Resource Collection.*

"Children's Health Care," the ACCH journal, and "ACCH Network" print reviews of books, videos, and films. A membership in ACCH makes these reviews and "The Directory of Resources" available to family resource librarians.

Bibliographies on medical subjects, parenting, the hospital experience, and other related topics can be provided by the public library. Occasionally, the public library turns to a Family Resource Collection for recommendations.

SPECIAL CONSIDERATION OF FICTION

When purchasing fiction for a Family Resource Collection, note the sources of medical expertise relied upon by the author. All fiction must be reviewed carefully by the librarian and by at least one

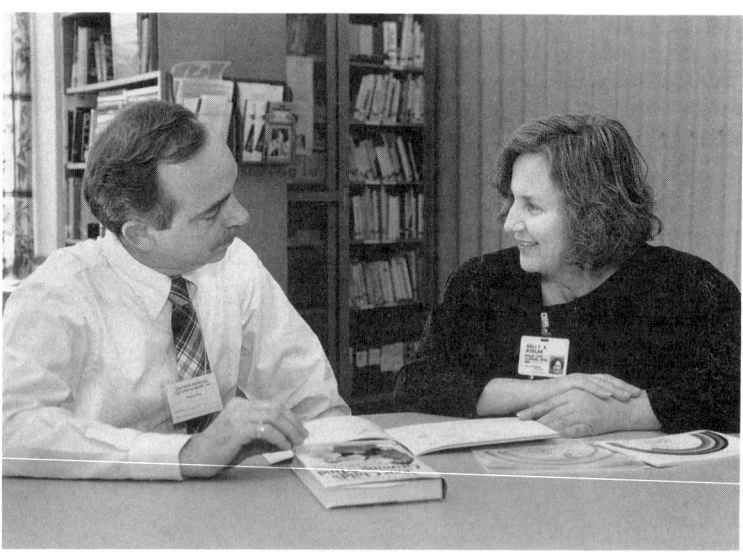

A parent and a child life specialist discuss a child's return to school.

medical staff member. Fiction authors may be tempted to over-dramatize, departing from medical reality and facts. *Growing Pains — Helping Children Deal with Everyday Problems through Reading* (Cuddigan) is a helpful resource.

SPECIAL CONSIDERATION OF CIRCULATION

So as to be as sure as possible that the "right book" gets into a parent's hands at the "right time," it is recommended that materials be circulated only through the librarian or other staff member. Sometimes, after careful conversation with the parent, the librarian learns that a child's diagnosis has not even been verified. "That's a good idea to wait," a parent said to the librarian. "Why should I scare myself when I may not need to?"

SPECIAL CONSIDERATION OF COLLECTION SIZE

While a variety of materials is desirable, the size of the collection is not the first consideration. Depth and quality are more important than quantity. Up-to-date materials are of prime importance. Generally, the best way to keep the collection updated is periodically to procure pamphlets and brochures from health agencies. Their content is subject to frequent revisions as recent findings and medical protocols are reported. Also, the time lapse between a pamphlet's preparation and printing is far shorter than it is for the publication of a book, where medical information can be outdated by the time the book hits the marketplace!

SPECIAL CONSIDERATION OF THE COLLECTION'S VALUE

Often, the value of the Family Resource Collection is most evident in a parent's remark: "If we had only had a book like this when our child was first injured." One parent said: "Fourteen years — and finally, here is information on my child's heart defect, even a diagram!" A mother of a disabled child told the librarian that, until she read the family support books, she assumed that there was something wrong with her that she felt guilty and alone.

Experiences like these are additional, convincing evidence of the need for and the value of a Family Resource Collection. The Resources section at the back of this book lists recommended basic titles for starting a Family Resource Collection.

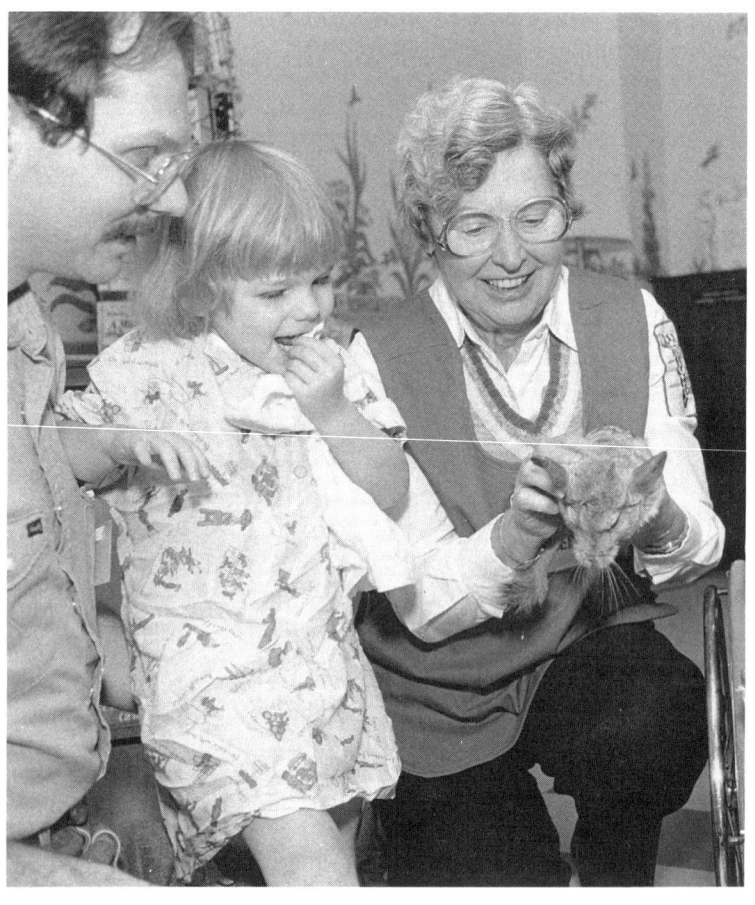

A zoo docent and a chinchilla visit Story Hour.   (Photo: Janet Century)

Chapter 13.

COMMUNITY OUTREACH:
A Two-Way Street

Community outreach is a two-way street in which many pediatric hospital library programs participate to one degree or another. The following text illustrates ways in which family resource libraries serve the greater community as well as ways in which the greater community serves the hospital's library program.

Some states have only one pediatric hospital; a few have none at all and are served by a pediatric facility in a neighboring state. In these instances, "community" can cover a very large area. Hospitals with far ranging patient services have an imperative to share informational materials and support networks through innovative programming.

This chapter offers a few profiles of family resource libraries with strong links to the larger community. It offers also profiles of strong community links to library programs. Only a few of the many services offered could be included here.

HOSPITAL RESOURCE LIBRARY OUTREACH TO THE COMMUNITY

Children's Hospital of Alabama, Birmingham, AL

The Comprehensive Health Educational Center for Kids (CHECK) provides information and programs to families, teachers, and child care providers throughout the state. A few of the programs offered are: Child Abuse Prevention; National "Safe Kids" Program to reduce accidental injuries and deaths; and program presentations on specific diseases with information provided by CHECK.

Phoenix Children's Hospital, Phoenix, AZ

The Emily Anderson Family Learning Center provides medical information to persons in the general community. The material is prepared according to individual needs and is disseminated through mailing packets that include a glossary of medical terms.

Children's Hospital Medical Center of Akron, Akron, OH
The Parent Coalition is based in Children's Hospital and co-operates with the hospital's Parent Library in distributing information. The Coalition serves as a partnership between parents and care providers for the preschool and school age disabled child in the larger community. In particular, the Coalition provides early interventions such as: medical referrals; information on education programs; and support group contacts.

Children's Hospital and Medical Center, Seattle, WA
Classes and programs offered by the Children's Resource Center are publicized through the "Good Growing Newsletter." The Children's Resource Line is manned by pediatric nurses, who answer questions on parenting and on children's illness and health. The Line is sponsored by a parent support group, public librarian, and hospital staff. The "Hospital Playkit" for children two-and-a-half to six years is available on a free loan basis to parents, day care providers, and preschool instructors.

COMMUNITY OUTREACH TO THE HOSPITAL LIBRARY

Public Library
Tampa, FL: The Tampa/Hillsborough Public Library System provides librarians who present story hours and book talks on a regular basis to five area pediatric hospitals. Librarian salaries are paid half by the hospital and half by the public library. The program is coordinated through the Florida Diagnostic and Learning Resources System at the University of South Florida (FDLRS/USF) Library Media Resources.

Phoenix, AZ: The Phoenix Public Library recognizes the Emily Anderson Family Learning Center as an "unofficial" branch. The Center's medical bibliography is on-line with the public library's data base.

Oklahoma City, OK: The Oklahoma State Department of Libraries cooperates with the Family Resource Center, Children's Hospital of Oklahoma in shared bibliographies and data bases.

Cleveland, OH: The Cuyahoga County Public Library System shares Summer Reading Club materials and ideas with the hospital library, Rainbow Babies and Childrens Hospital.

San Francisco, CA: The San Francisco Public Library recruits, trains, and supports volunteers who take part in the "Book Buddies" program. Volunteers read aloud to children in six area hospitals.

Carson, CA: The County of Los Angeles Public Libraries funds staff and programming for the Consumer Health Information Program and Services at Carson Regional Library in conjunction with the Harbor UCLA Medical Center. Programs include "Tel Med", prerecorded tapes to answer telephoned medical questions, and mailings in response to requests for information. Specific subjects of interest may be child abuse, medical subjects, physician referrals, and support groups.

OTHER COMMUNITY SUPPORTS FOR HOSPITAL LIBRARY PROGRAMS

Donations of new books provided by
 Book store owners
 Free-lance and staff book reviewers
 School library jobbers
 Publisher warehouses
 Awards committee members
 Reviewers of materials for publishers of book bibliographies
  for children

Program Volunteers — a New Source
 Corporate volunteerism is a growing concept, exemplified by Apple Computer and Ampex Corporations. Employee volunteers read aloud to pediatric patients at The Lucile Salter Packard Children's Hospital at Stanford, CA.

Library Program Enrichment for Young Patients
 Volunteer docents from the Cleveland Metroparks Zoo present educational "small animal" programs during Story Hours and, afterwards, take the animals onto the patient floors for children unable to leave their rooms.
 "Young Audiences," a national organization with local and regional chapters, presents high quality programs for children in music, dance, and theater, including puppetry and storytelling. Payments for performances are provided by family foundations and corporate gifts.

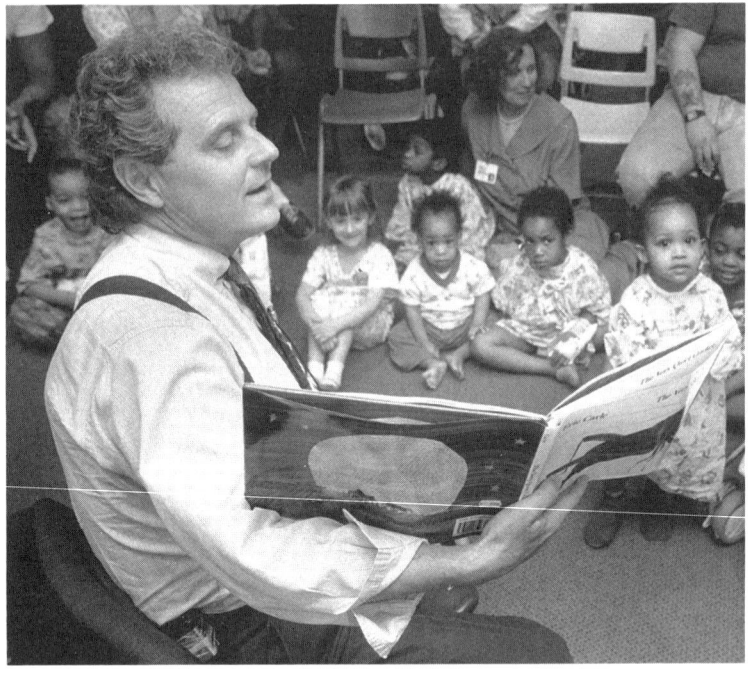

To help celebrate "National Library Week," a TV news anchorman reads aloud to young patients.   (Photo by Images)

Various opportunities to help promote reading and library use exist in pediatric hospitals. "Celebrity Readers," who are holders of public office, entertainers, and media newscasters read aloud in a number of hospitals to promote "National Library Week" and "Children's Book Week."

A unique read-a-long between young patients at the Shriners Children's Hospital and members of the University of South Florida basketball team was held "on court" in Tampa, FL.

AN AFTERTHOUGHT

This chapter is representative of only a few family resource libraries with outreach commitments both to the community and from the community. Readers interested in getting in touch with directors of these library programs and other ones can contact the National Center for Family Centered Care at ACCH: (301) 654-6549.

Chapter 14.

ESPECIALLY FOR FAMILIES

Nearly all aspects of library programming empower parents, grandparents, and siblings in a family-centered care environment. The following information may be of interest to families of hospitalized children.

BOOKS

Before a hospital stay, preparation through books is recommended as long as the information is presented honestly. At least, your child becomes aware through the story that other children have had similar hospital experiences and have returned to home and school. There is strength in knowing that.

While a book like *Curious George Goes to the Hospital* (Rey) is not realistic, the humor in it is appreciated by children who are already hospitalized. That your child laughs is reason enough to share the book with him.

Often the child who has an emergency admission will need additional support and some "talking through" the experience. The librarian can be helpful by giving out a hospital experience book and other pertinent information.

READING ALOUD

While your child is in the hospital, read aloud to her at every opportunity. Reading aloud is not only comforting to the child, but to the parent as well. Stress levels can be significantly lowered for both of you.

In addition, reading aloud in a medical setting is something parents do best. By reading to your child, you are communicating

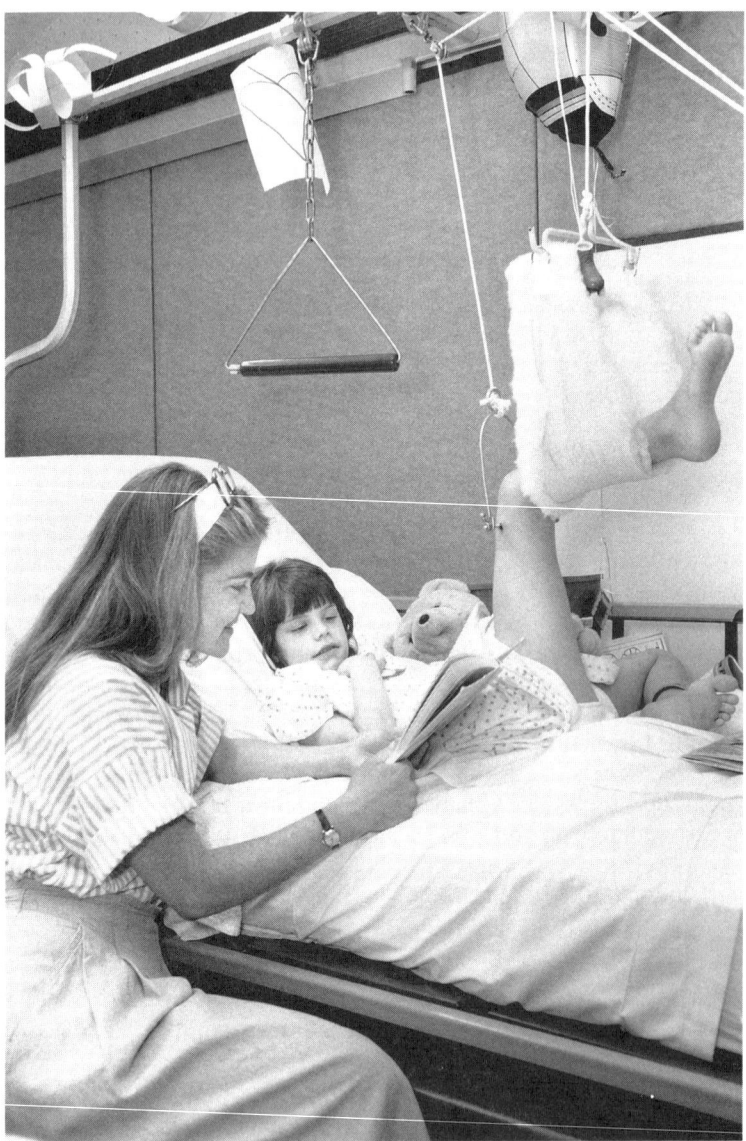

A parent reads to her child in the orthopedic x-ray corridor.

with her. The sound of your voice is reassuring. The very young child may not be able to comprehend a story, but he does recognize a parent's voice. Parents unable to stay with their children will frequently tape books for their children to listen to during the parents' absence.

When you read aloud, you and your child are experiencing the warmth of an intimate time without the demands of job, household responsibilities, and other persons in the family. "In the long run, the only things of lasting value you can give a child is your time and the memories of the time you shared together."[1]

Often, your child's frustration at being unable to respond to your conversation or to initiate any disappears when he needs only to listen.

Sit close to your child as you read. She needs you and you need her.

As your child's health improves, you are helping to maintain and build upon her cognitive and verbal skills.

The librarian, child life specialist, or other staff members can read in your absence. Volunteers read aloud too.

In addition to reading in a child's hospital room, playroom, or library, parents have read aloud to their children during premedication before treatments, in the holding area prior to surgery, during imaging procedures, and in the recovery room. Parents can read aloud any place they go with their children.

If your child has a lengthy confinement in the hospital or at home, keep her in touch with the changing world outside her window by reading her seasonal titles.

If, because of injury or illness, your child has been unresponsive, but shows response during your reading aloud, pass on the information to the primary care nurse so that the observations can be entered in your child's chart.

BIBLIOTHERAPY

Often without realizing it, parents and their children practice informal bibliotherapy when both read a book and talk about it. "The characters in the book, since they are not real people, can be discussed without fear of hurting anyone's feelings or of being hurt in return."[2] Sharing responses and ideas in this way creates another bond between parent and child and can lead to new insights.

STORY HOUR

Try to stay with your child in Story Hour. It will be a time you can enjoy together that takes you both away from the hospital room.

If you cannot stay, don't leave abruptly. Some children will be so worried that you are gone that they cannot really listen. Consult with the librarian and assure your child that you will return at the scheduled end of Story Hour. Volunteers and other adults will be with your child.

Sometimes the Story Hour program can lead to follow-up reading or activities back on the floor or at home. One mother said that her seriously ill child's problem of what to give her family members for Christmas had been solved by the Story Hour activity of decorating gingerbread boy cookies.

FAMILY RESOURCE COLLECTION

Use the Family Resource Collection, for it is designed primarily for you. Sometimes a book you find helpful is worth sharing with other parents. The librarian is always happy to receive suggestions of titles that can be of further support to families.

Understanding what your doctor has told you about your child's illness and its treatment can become clearer when you read about it. Ask the librarian for any available materials. If further information raises more questions, write down those questions to ask your child's doctor or nurse.

The Family Resource Collection should also inform you about parent support groups, parent networks, and various community agencies providing health and social services. In addition, many collections include materials for siblings and friends, classmates and teachers.

BOOK CART

Take advantage of the librarian's presence on the floor. If your child's hospital stay is extensive, you might want to ask the librarian to track down some specific information for you or your child.

At all times, the librarian is open to you and your child's suggestions of authors, subjects, and titles for the general book collection. One librarian carries a note pad for this very purpose.

GOING HOME

When your child goes home, much of what she has experienced goes home with her. She may be fretful and upset for a few days. Rereading some of the hospital experience books may help her to resolve her feelings. Most public libraries include hospital experience books in the children's section.

Talk with her and give her time to adjust to the return home. Reading familiar books in a familiar space helps to reassure her that she is home again.

Sometimes, fathers find it difficult to help in a situation involving their child's hospitalization. Read to your young child. These picture book titles are recommended:

Owl Moon (Yolen)
No Nap (Bunting)
The Stupids Step Out (Allard)
Daddy Makes the Best Spaghetti (Hines)
Patrick's Dinosaurs (Carrick)

Some of these books highlight the relationship between father and child.

In addition to the above titles for the young child, preschool and school age children will enjoy sharing nonfiction books with fathers:

Train Song (Siebert)
Night Sky (Barrett, N. S.)
Whales (Berger)
Sharks (Berger)
Beacons of Light (Gibbons)
Digging Up Dinosaurs (Aliki)
The Story of the Statue of Liberty (Maestro)
Teammates (Golenbock)

Learning something together is its own kind of support and is nurturing in a hospital environment.

GRANDPARENTS ARE SPECIAL

Even without trying very hard, grandparents have a special relationship with grandchildren. A stress in the family, such as a grandchild's hospitalization, is an opportunity to strengthen a mutually nurturing relationship.

Sensing that grandparents are one step removed from the situation, grandchildren sometimes confide their worries and fears to a grandparent and seek support and reassurance.

One way for a grandparent to support and reassure is to read aloud. Grandchildren like to hear stories about grandparents' own childhood. Fortunately, today there are many such books published. *When I Was Young in the Mountains* (Rylant), *In Coal Country* (Hendershot), and *Home Place* (Dragonwagon) are three such books.

It is important too that books read by grandparents have a view into the future. *Family Farm* (Locker) and *Grandma's Promise* (Moore) project into the years ahead.

Although grandparents can experience the "double whammy" of observing the discomfort of a grandchild and their own child, they can sometimes be persuaded to read an amusing story in a far from amusing situation. *Amelia Bedelia* (Parish) in all titles, *Henry and Mudge* (Rylant) in all titles, and the Henry Huggins and Ramona books (Cleary) are examples of just a few authors with a gift for sparking contagious laughter.

Books proliferate about the bond between grandparent and grandchild:

That Sky, That Rain (Otto) Knowing that a rainstorm approaches, a grandfather tends to the farm animals with his granddaughter. When the clouds burst, they share the magic of a storm.

The Patchwork Quilt (Flournoy) Through the piecing and stitching of a patchwork quilt, a special relationship grows between a grandmother, mother, and grandaughter.

Grampa's Face (Greenfield) Bold, pastel illustrations depict the story of a little girl's love and sensitivity for her grandfather. An example of the importance of good communication in overcoming anxiety.

Come a Tide (Lyon) A lighthearted, folksy look at a March flood in the Kentucky mountains. Grandma predicts it and the rest of the mountain folks react with good humor and hard work.

Because parents are involved in trying to meet their child's daily needs and treatments, less preoccupied grandparents sometimes take over the ongoing commitment to maintaining reading skills. Books by the Berenstains, Lobel, and Eastman are always popular.

Other times, grandparents are the ones who bring children to Story Hour.

Sometimes, a grandparent's promise of a follow-up to a shared story offers an element of hope and affirmation, e.g., "When you get home, we'll make the cake in this story" or "We'll take a trip there, you and I."

Grandparents have a unique status. By their very presence in the hospital, they offer their grandchildren and their "own children a sense of security and reassurance during times of stress."[3]

The gift of a book sent by a distant grandparent can create a special bond. You will be helped to "be there" with your grandchild even though you are many miles away.

SIBLINGS ARE SPECIAL

Brothers and sisters have been called the "forgotten ones." Shunted off to other members of the extended family or alone much of the time, they suffer from separation as well as from feelings of jealousy, guilt, and anger.

Picture books and realistic fiction can help siblings recognize that other siblings have shared the same situation and feelings, and have survived the ordeal. The following titles are recommended for siblings:

Summer of the Swans (Byars) brain damage
C.F. In His Corner (Radley) cystic fibrosis
I Have a Sister, My Sister is Deaf (Peterson)
Welcome Home, Jellybean (Shyer) developmental delay
A Summer to Die (Lowry) death due to cancer
Inside Out (Martin, A.) autism
Our Brother Has Down's Syndrome (Cairo)
My Sister's Special (Prall) brain damage
I Can Say No (Sanford) drug addiction
I Wish I Was Sick Too! (Brandenberg)
Finding a Way — Living with Exceptional Brothers and Sisters
   (Rosenberg) asthma, spina bifida, diabetes
Waiting for Baby Joe (Collins, P.) prematurity
My Brother Steven is Retarded (Sobol, H.)
And Don't Bring Jeremy (Levinson) neurological impairment
Losing Someone You Love: When a Brother or Sister Dies
   (Richter)
Where's Buddy? (Roy) diabetes
I'm the Big Sister Now (Emmert) cerebral palsy

Having a child in the hospital is a stressful situation, but many families find that by taking advantage of psychosocial supports, such as the library program, they can turn a traumatic experience into one of growth and affirmation.

MOM

Every day I thought of you

Every day my dreams came true

I missed you

and you'll never know

about the nights.

I felt sorrow,

but you're back

and here to stay.

Never again will I stray

for I found a place

to keep my love,

a special place from up above.

And now we've made a brand

new start

and my special place

is in your heart.

Poem by a young patient

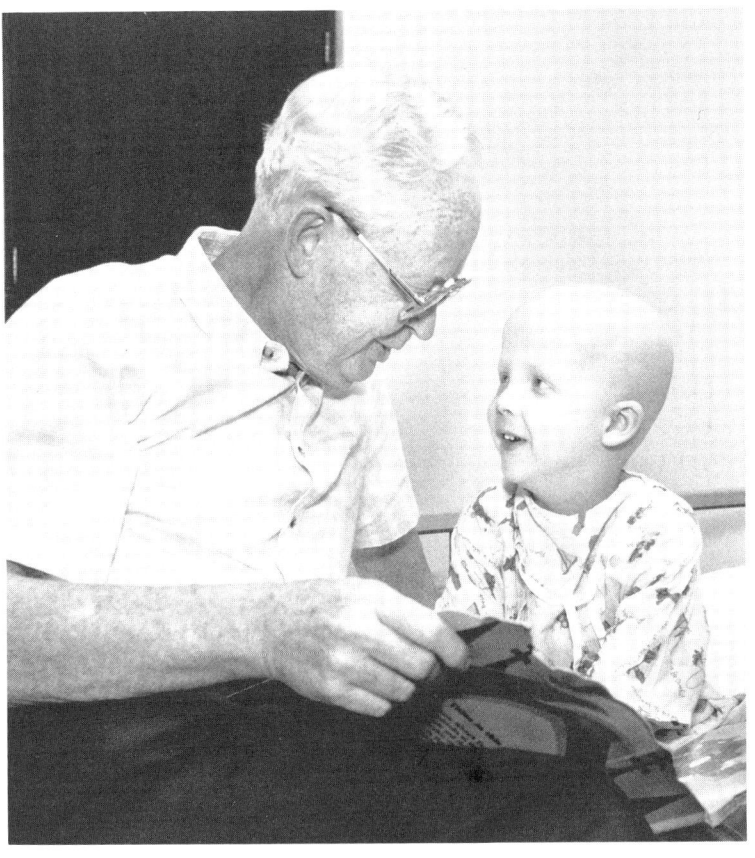

Grandparents are special readers.

Chapter 15.

ESPECIALLY FOR LIBRARIANS:
Professional and Volunteer Professional

Many pediatric hospitals with a library program are served by volunteer librarians — sometimes by librarians who are retired from schools or public libraries, but more often by lay volunteers with an enthusiasm for the work. Other hospitals have librarians with all ranges of professional background, skills, and experiences. Sometimes a hospital staff member takes on the responsibilities.

Whatever the librarian's background, the following requirements seem essential:

Communication skills
Willingness to be involved with patient/family needs
Resource skills — especially information retrieval
Knowledge of literature for children and young adults
Self-motivation and initiative
Flexibility to adapt traditional library services to meet the
   special needs of hospitalized children

A FEW INSIGHTS ABOUT THE JOB

Positives: As a librarian, you are a known quantity. Children and their families relate easily to you. Much of the programming is familiar. A mother said: "My child was so disappointed he had to come to the hospital yesterday and miss Story Hour at the public library. And now, Story Hour's here!"

In addition, many of the collection materials will be familiar. Often, parents will borrow books they remember as children. A father pulled *The Red Badge of Courage* (Crane) from the shelf and said, "I never had a chance to read this."

On spotting a new book on display, a child said: "I'm on the wait list for this book at school — and now I've got it!"

The existence of a library with active programming can help to normalize the hospital experience by reducing strangeness and offering materials that entertain, inform, and support the child and his family. Librarians can offer children a certain stabilizing influence in their lives.

Negatives: A hospital librarian's job can be a solitary one. Although volunteers are a source of mutual support, a sharing relationship with one or two staff members offers a chance to "rap" when stress levels are high. A pediatric hospital can be an emotionally challenging environment for everyone.

Friendships within the public library sector and attendance at local and regional conferences can be professionally supportive and can also assuage a sense of isolation. Further support can come from membership in ACCH, providing opportunities for networking with fellow hospital librarians.

Less easy to deal with is a hospital librarian's frustration with bureaucracy; and, in some pediatric settings, the low priority placed on library services.

A FEW INSIGHTS ABOUT THE CHILDREN

It goes without saying that, outwardly, hospitalized children are not the same as children in a normal environment. This is especially noticeable during a Story Hour program. Unless they are soon to be discharged or are siblings visiting, many of the children will be low in energy. Some will be distracted, medicated and/or perhaps withdrawn. Their participation in the program will be more often receptive than expressive. There may be disappointing Story Hours when it is unclear whether any child was reached. After one such session, the librarian was surprised later to hear a child say to her: "I know you. You told us the story about the windup mouse!" Someone was listening!

Though the librarian must work hard to elicit responses, it is important to try to do so. Often a child will then interact with the group and gain in confidence and self-esteem.

A hospital librarian who takes the same Preschool Story Hour program to a community preschool will experience a hilarious and excited response. Hospitalized children may simply watch the puppet show; usually well children interact verbally with the puppets. A hospitalized child focuses well on the flannel board, but must be encouraged on a one-on-one basis to move around a felt figure on the board held in front of him; well children surge forward to do so.

Especially in hospital Story Hour, books can act as an agent for the relief of anxiety. During a birthday story, a child started sobbing and left the library. Afterward, he confided that he was afraid he would not be home for his own birthday. Learning of his anxiety, the librarian assured him that, at home or in the hospital, he would have a party.

The librarian showed a picture of a racoon and a child burst forth with: "My grandmother and I hate rats. We found one sleeping in my mother's shoe." This outburst offered the opportunity to explain carefully the difference between a rat and a racoon and to give the parent an opportunity to talk over with her child an understandable fear.

FOR THE PROFESSIONAL LIBRARIAN

Simple color coding of materials can seem "unprofessional"; book circulation and return may seem haphazard and unaccountable; maintaining the collection and ordering new materials may seem too low on the priority list.

But color coding enables patients, families, staff, and volunteers to locate and identify materials most easily; book circulation and return operate in a manner most conducive for reaching the majority of children and their families; and maintaining the collection and ordering new materials can be assigned to volunteers under a librarian's direction.

FOR THE VOLUNTEER PROFESSIONAL

In initiating a library program, it works best sometimes to start with a single service, e.g., reading aloud to individual patients, developing a Family Resource Collection, offering a weekly Story Hour, or providing book cart services.

The public library should be in a position to help. "Outreach" programs may offer storytelling services especially for the school age child. Plentiful materials for use in a Preschool Story Hour and an uncritical audience make it surprisingly easy for volunteer/ professional librarians to provide story hours for preschoolers.

Until you have funds available for major purchases, the public library can also be a source of materials — books, flannel board stories, filmstrips, and music tapes.

Even with the help of this publication and numerous other titles listed under Resources, moving somewhat slowly and consolidating your gains and support within and outside of the hospital will assure a more permanent success.

PART OF THE TEAM

Hospital librarians are a part of the team. As a resource person, the librarian is a team member who reaches out to serve all segments of the hospital population. Through access to published materials, she may be the one to serve as a catalyst for new plans and ideas requiring information retrieval.

It is important that she publicize the library's collection and services, not only to the patients and families, but also to the various departments. As with other facets of the library program, promotion and reminders are necessary: posters in prominent places, memos, publicity in in-house newsletters, and meetings with staff.

The Hospital Public School Program

The hospital school is one of the programs most frequently served by the library. The rationale for a hospital school with certified teachers is that children benefit from their involvement in schoolwork: "It not only gives them continuity in their learning, but it also brings a sense of normalcy to the daily routine."[1] Particularly for the chronically ill child, it can sometimes make the difference between passing and failing the school year.

In addition, the library can provide motivational factors for getting well and for getting on with school and with life goals.

The library is a source of primary materials for school assignments and of secondary resources for basic curriculum units. The librarian can further help the student by assisting her in making information phone calls to museum librarians and curators. Sometimes, older patients require special materials as resources for lengthy term papers. One student needed biographies of Adolf Hitler borrowed from the public library.

Easy readers augment early reading skills. Many fiction titles fulfill a majority of class reading assignments.

The poetry writing program supports the language arts. During poetry time, the child learns poetic forms, acquires techniques of self-expression, and reads some poetry. Most importantly, all written efforts are encouraged and appreciated.

The library space can support the school program by providing a place to study, to obtain books for enjoyment and for school assignments, to spend time in a normalized environment where socialization occurs, and an opportunity to relate to a librarian and teacher who are nonmedical persons.

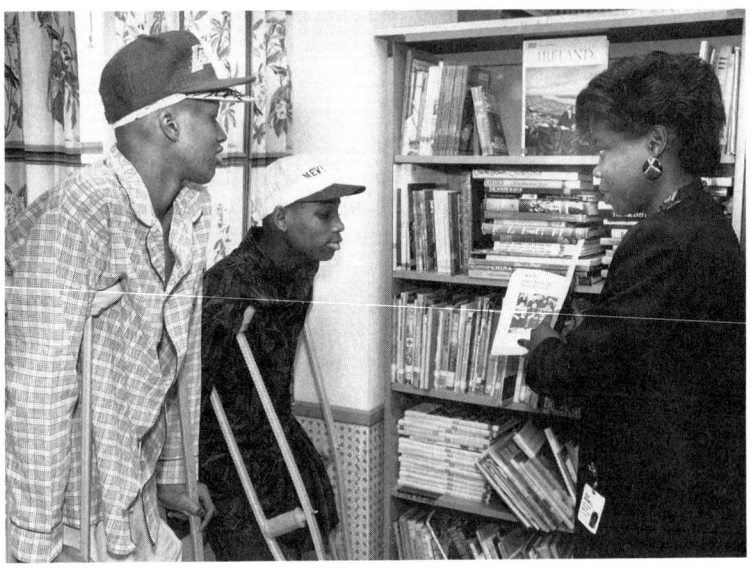

Students in the hospital school are assisted in locating resource materials.

Other Departments

Networking with and supporting hospital personnel is vital. In order to operate the library program as a supportive adjunct to the hospital's multidisciplinary team, the librarian must be accessible, alert to needs, and responsive to requests from all staff members.

Conclusion

As the years have passed, the patient/family librarian has become a more accepted member of the medical health care team. There is still much work to be done.

In order to achieve ultimate acceptance, we must continue our commitment to professional development and to imagination in adaptive programming. We must also support a network of fellow librarians and ever higher standards of work and materials.

Along with other caregivers, patient/family librarians share concern for the whole child, for an affirmation of his wellness, and for a widening of his vision and the enrichment of his spirit. We believe that books offering identifiable characters, accurate information, and passages that resonate in a child's own experience make a difference in the lives of hospitalized children.

> *Many things can wait. The child cannot.*
> *To him we cannot say tomorrow. His name is today.*

Gabriela Mistral, Chilean Writer
Winner of Nobel Prize for Literature, 1945

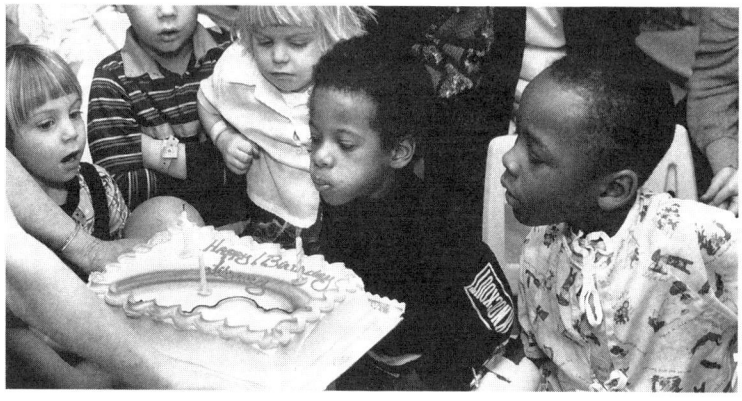

A Story Hour celebration of the library's birthday.

Notes

Introduction

1. Emma Plank, *Working with Children in Hospitals*. (Chicago, IL: Year Book Medical Publishers 1971), p. 1.

2. Plank, p.1.

3. "Statements of Policy for the Care of Children and Families in Health Care Settings". (Washington, DC: Association for the Care of Children's Health, 1977).

Chapter 2: Building the Collection for the Hospitalized Child

1. Walter de la Mare, *Bells and Grass: A Book of Rhymes* (New York: Viking, 1963), p.9.

2. Frank Self, "Choosing for Children Under Three." *CBC Features* (New York: Children's Book Council, 1987).

3. Natalie Babbitt, "Protecting Children's Literature," *The Horn Book Magazine*, November-December 1990, pp. 701-702.

4. Claudia Lepman-Logan, "Books in the Classroom: Moral Choices in Literature," *The Horn Book Magazine*, January-February 1989, p.110.

5. Jim Trelease, *The New Read-Aloud Handbook* (New York: Penguin, 1989), p.55.

6. Elizabeth Speare, "The Survival Story," *The Horn Book Magazine*, March-April 1988, p.172.

7. Bernie Siegel,M.D., *Love, Medicine and Miracles* (New York: Harper & Row, 1986), p.144.

8. Leland Jacobs, "Getting the Most Out of Humor," *Teaching K-8*, April 1989, p.30.

Chapter 3: Offering a Story Hour for Toddlers, Preschoolers, and Siblings

1. Jane Healy, From a speech delivered at Hathaway Brown School, Cleveland, OH, November 7, 1990.

2. Jane Healy, *Endangered Minds: Why Our Children Don't Think* (New York: Simon & Schuster, 1990), p.104.

3. Jane Healy, *Your Child's Growing Mind* (New York: Doubleday, 1987), p.160.

4. Judy Nichols, *Storytimes for Two-Year-Olds* (Chicago: American Library Association, 1988), p.8.

Chapter 5: Offering a Story Hour for School Age Children and Siblings

1. Bernice Cullinan et al., *Literature and the Child* (New York: Harcourt Brace Jovanovich, 1981), p.19.

2. Norma Fox Mazer, "Growing Up with Stories," *Top of the News*, Vol.41, No. 2, Winter 1985, p.165.

3. Karen Olness, M.D., Rainbow Babies and Childrens Hospital, Cleveland, OH, April 1991.

4. Dorothy de Wit, *Children's Faces Looking Up: Program Building for the Storyteller* (Chicago: The American Library Association, 1979), p.29.

5. Natalie Babbitt, "Protecting Children's Literature," *The Horn Book Magazine*, November-December, 1990, p.703.

Chapter 8: Library Services to Children with Special Needs

1. Susan Kleinberg, *Educating the Chronically Ill Child* (London: An Aspen Publication, 1982), p.146.

2. Jane Healy, *Endangered Minds: Why Our Children Don't Think*, p.63.

3. Healy, p.93.

4. Jean A. Pardeck and John T. Pardeck, *Books for Early Childhood: A Developmental Perspective* (Westport, CT: Greenwood Press, 1988), p.9.

Chapter 10: Bibliotherapy with Hospitalized Children

1 Doris Robinson, From a lecture given at Lakewood Public Library, Lakewood, OH, February 16, 1991.

2. Joanne Bernstein and Masha Rudman, *Books to Help Children Cope with Separation and Loss: An Annotated Bibliography* (New York: Bowker, 1989), p.36.

3. Bernstein and Rudman, p.36.

4. Joan Fassler, *Helping Children Cope: Mastering Stress Through Books and Stories* (New York: Macmillan, 1978), p.152.

5. Katherine Paterson, "Living in a Peaceful World," *The Horn Book Magazine*, January-February, 1991, p.34.

6. Alan Rosenthal, "How Fantasy Helps Kids Grow," *Parents*, May 1988, p.92.

7. Bernstein and Rudman, p.39.

Chapter 11: Poetry Writing in a Pediatric Setting

1. Doris Robinson, Lakewood Public Library, February 16, 1991.

2. Millicent Lenz, "The Search for Wholeness: When Children Write Poetry," *Children Today*, May-June, 1981, p.7.

Chapter 12: A Family Resource Collection

1. Robin B. Thomas, "Research Commentary: A Foundation for Clinical Family Assessment," *Children's Health Care*, Vol. 19, No. 4, Fall 1990, p. 247.

Chapter 14: Especially for Families

1. Jim Trelease, *The New Read-Aloud Handbook*, p.XXIV.

2. Doris Robinson, "Talking It Out: The Use of Books in Discussion for Developmental Bibliotherapy with Children," *Top of the News*, Vol 41, No. 2, 1985, p.151.

3. Irene Springer, "What Every Grandparent Should Know" — An Interview with T. Berry Brazelton, M.D., *Parade*, March 1990, p.16.

Chapter 15: Especially for Librarians — Professional and Volunteer Professional

1. Gertrude Morrow, *Helping Chronically Ill Children in School* (West Nyack, NY:Parker Publishing Co., 1985), p.98.

Bibliography of Recommended Children's Books

Aliki. *Digging Up Dinosaurs.* New York: Harper, 1988.

Allard, Harry. *Miss Nelson is Missing!* Boston: Houghton Mifflin, 1977.

—.*The Stupids Step Out.* Boston: Houghton Mifflin, 1977.

Anderson, Lena. *Stina.* New York: Greenwillow, 1989.

Aragon, Jane Chelsea. *Winter Harvest.* Boston: Little, Brown, 1989.

Asch, Frank. *Goodbye House.* New York: Simon & Schuster, 1989.

—.*Just Like Daddy.* New York: Simon & Schuster, 1980.

—.*Mooncake.* New York: Simon & Schuster, 1983.

Atwater, Richard. *Mr. Popper's Penguins.* Boston: Little, Brown, 1938.

Avi. *The True Confessions of Charlotte Doyle.* New York: Orchard Books, 1990.

Ballard, Robert D. *Exploring the Titanic.* New York: Scholastic, 1988.

Bang, Molly. *Ten, Nine, Eight.* New York: Greenwillow, 1983.

Barrett, Judi. *Cloudy with a Chance of Meatballs.* New York: Macmillan, 1978.

Barrett, N.S. *Night Sky.* New York: Franklin Watts, 1985.

Barrie, J.M. *Peter Pan.* Plattsburgh, NY: Tundra Books, 1988.

Barton, Byron. *Bones, Bones, Dinosaur Bones.* New York: Harper, 1990.

Bauer, Marian Dan. *On My Honor.* New York: Ticknor & Fields, 1986.

Bawden, Nina. *William Tell.* New York: Lothrop, 1981.

Berger, Gilda. *Sharks.* New York: Doubleday, 1987.

—.*Whales.* New York: Doubleday, 1987.

Blos, Joan W. *Martin's Hats.* New York: Morrow, 1984.

Blume, Judy. *Superfudge.* New York: Dutton, 1980.

—.*Tales of a Fourth Grade Nothing.* New York: Dutton, 1972.

Boden, Alice. *The Field of Buttercups.* New York: H.Z. Walck, 1974.

Bonnici, Peter. *The First Rains.* Minneapolis, MN: Carolrhoda Books, 1985.

Books for World Explorers. Washington, DC: National Geographic Society.

Booth, David. *'Til All the Stars Have Fallen.* New York: Viking, 1990.

Bornstein, Ruth. *A Beautiful Seashell.* New York: Harper, 1990.

Boulton, Sir Harold. *All Through the Night.* Nashville, TN: Abingdon, 1988.

Brandenberg, Franz. *I Wish I Was Sick Too!* New York: Greenwillow, 1976.

Brett, Jan. *The Mitten.* New York: Putnam, 1990.

Brinckloe, Julie. *Fireflies!* New York: Macmillan, 1975.

Brown, Marc. *Hand Rhymes.* New York: Dutton, 1985.

Brown, Margaret Wise. *The Big Red Barn.* New York: Harper, 1989
—.*Goodnight, Moon.* New York: Harper, 1947.
—.*Home for a Bunny.* New York: Western, 1983.
—.*The Runaway Bunny.* New York: Harper, 1942.

Brown, Ruth. *The Big Sneeze.* New York: Lothrop, 1985.

Bunting, Eve. *How Many Days to America?* Boston: Houghton Mifflin, 1990.
—.*Mother's Day Mice.* New York: Clarion, 1986.
—.*No Nap.* Boston: Houghton Mifflin, 1989.
—.*Our Sixth Grade Sugar Babies.* New York: Harper, 1990.
—.*St. Patrick's Day in the Morning.* Boston: Houghton Mifflin, 1980.
—.*The Valentine Bears.* Boston: Houghton Mifflin, 1983.
—.*The Wednesday Surprise.* Boston: Houghton Mifflin, 1990.

Burningham, John McKintosh. *Hey! Get Off Our Train!* New York: Crown, 1990.
—.*Mr. Gumpy's Outing.* New York: Holt, Henry & Co., 1990.

Burstein, Fred. *Anna's Rain.* New York: Orchard Books, 1990.

Burton, Virginia Lee. *The Little House.* Boston: Houghton Mifflin, 1978.

Butler, Dorothy. *My Brown Bear Barney.* New York: Greenwillow, 1989.

Byars, Betsy C. *Bingo Brown and the Language of Love.* New York: Viking, 1989.
—.*A Blossom Promise.* New York: Delacorte, 1987.
—.*Summer of the Swans.* New York: Viking, 1970.

Cairo, Shelley. *Our Brother Has Down's Syndrome.* Toronto: Annick Press, Ltd., 1985.

Cameron, Ann. *The Stories Julian Tells.* New York: Pantheon, 1981.

Campbell, Rod. *Dear Zoo.* New York: Viking, 1982.

Carle, Eric. *The Very Busy Spider.* New York: Philomel Books, 1984.
—.*The Very Hungry Caterpillar.* New York: Philomel Books, 1979.
—.*The Very Quiet Cricket.* New York: Philomel Books, 1990.

Carrick, Carol. *Lost in the Storm.* New York: Seabury Press, 1974.
—.*Patrick's Dinosaurs.* Boston: Houghton Mifflin, 1983.
—.*A Rabbit for Easter.* New York: Greenwillow, 1979
—.*What Happened to Patrick's Dinosaurs?* New York: Ticknor & Fields, 1986.

Christian, Mary Blount. *Swamp Monsters.* New York: Dial, 1983.

Cleary, Beverly. *Henry Huggins.* New York: Morrow, 1957.
—.*Ramona the Pest.* New York: Morrow, 1968.

Clifton, Lucille. *Amifika*. New York: Dutton, 1977.

Coerr, Eleanor. *The Josefina Story Quilt*. New York: Harper, 1986.

Cohen, Miriam. *When Will I Read?* New York: Greenwillow, 1977.

Cole, Joanna. *Get Well Clown-Arounds!* New York: Crown, 1987.

——. *The Magic School Bus: Inside the Human Body*. New York: Scholastic, 1989.

Collins, Pat L. *Waiting for Baby Joe*. Niles, IL: Whitman, 1990.

Conford, Ellen. *If This Is Love, I'll Take Spaghetti*. New York: Macmillan, 1983.

Crane, Stephen. *The Red Badge of Courage*. West Haven, CT: Pendulum, Press, 1973.

Crews, Donald. *Freight Train*. New York: Greenwillow, 1978.

Cromwell, Liz. *Finger Frolics*. Livonia, MI: Partner Press, 1976.

Curtis, Gavin. *Grandma's Baseball*. New York: Crown, 1990.

Dahl, Roald. *The B.F.G.* New York: Farrar, 1989.

Daly, Niki. *Not So Fast, Songololo*. New York: Macmillan, 1986.

Dancing Tepees. Edited by Virginia H. Sneve. New York: Holiday, 1989.

Daugherty, James. *Andy and the Lion*. New York: Viking, 1938.

DeClements, Barthe. *Nothing's Fair in Fifth Grade*. New York: Viking, 1981.

Delacre, Lulu. *Arroz Con Leche*. New York: Scholastic, 1989.

Delton, Judy. *I'm Telling You Now*. New York: Dutton, 1983.

dePaola, Tomie. *The Legend of the Indian Paintbrush*. New York: Putnam, 1988.

de Regniers, Beatrice. *A Week in the Life of Best Friends*. New York: Atheneum, 1986.

Dodge, Mary Mapes. *Hans Brinker or the Silver Skates*. New York: Scholastic, 1988.

Domanska, Jania. *The Turnip*. New York: Macmillan, 1969.

Dragonwagon, Crescent. *Home Place*. New York: Macmillan, 1990.

Drescher, Joan. *My Mother's Getting Married Again*. New York: Dial, 1986.

Dyer, Jane. *Moo, Moo, Peekaboo!* New York: Random House, 1986.

Eastman, P.D. *Are You My Mother?* New York: Random House, 1986.

Ekker, Ernest A. *What Is Beyond the Hill?* New York: Harper, 1986.

Emmert, Michelle. *I'm the Big Sister Now*. Niles, IL: Whitman, 1989.

Ende, Michael. *The Neverending Story*. New York: Doubleday, 1983.

Ernst, Lisa Campbell. *The Bee*. New York: Lothrop, 1986.

Esbensen, Barbara. *The Star Maiden*. Boston: Little, Brown, 1988.

Fisher, Aileen. *Out in the Dark and Daylight*. New York: Harper, 1980.

Flack, Marjorie. *Angus and the Cat*. New York: Doubleday, 1989.

——. *Ask Mr. Bear*. New York: Macmillan, 1932.

Florian, Douglas. *A Summer Day*. New York: Grenwillow, 1988.

Flournoy, Valerie. *The Patchwork Quilt*. New York: Dial, 1985.

Fowler, Richard. *Mr. Little's Noisy Car.*
New York: Putnam, 1986.

Fowler, Susi. *When Summer Ends.* New
York: Greenwillow, 1989.

Fox, Mem. *Hattie and the Fox.* New
York: Bradbury Press, 1988.

Freedman, Russell. *Lincoln: A
Photobiography.* New York:
Ticknor & Fields, 1987.

Freeman, Don. *Corduroy.* New York:
Viking, 1968.
—.*A Pocket for Corduroy.* New York:
Viking, 1978.

Frost, Robert. *Stopping By the Woods
on a Snowy Evening.* New York:
Dutton, 1978.
—.*The Road Not Taken.* New York:
Holt, Rinehart, 1985.

Fujikawa, Gyo. *Baby Mother Goose.*
New York: Random House, 1989.

Galdone, Paul. *Androcles and the Lion.*
New York: McGraw-Hill, 1970.
—.*The Gingerbread Boy.* Boston:
Houghton Mifflin, 1983.
—.*Jack and the Beanstalk.* Boston:
Houghton Mifflin, 1982.
—.*The Monkey and the Crocodile.* New
York: Ticknor & Fields, 1987.

Gauch, Patricia L. *Christina Katerina
and the Great Bear Train.* New
York: Putnam, 1990.

George, Jean Craighead. *My Side of the
Mountain.* New York: Dutton, 1988.
—.*On the Far Side of the Mountain.*
New York: Dutton, 1990.

Gibbons, Gail. *Beacons of Light.* New
York: Morrow, 1990.
—.*Dinosaurs.* New York: Holiday
House, 1987.

Ginsburg, Mirra. *Four Brave Sailors.*
New York: Greenwillow, 1987.

Glenn, Mel. *Class Dismissed! High
School Poems.* New York: Ticknor
& Fields, 1982.

Goennel, Heidi. *If I Were a Penguin.*
Boston: Little, Brown, 1989.
—.*Seasons.* Boston: Little, Brown,
1986.

Golenbock, Peter. *Teammates.* New
York: Harcourt, 1990.

Gray, Nigel. *A Country Far Away.* New
York: Orchard Books, 1989.

Grayson, Marion. *Let's Do Fingerplays.*
Bridgeport, CT: Luce, 1962.

Green, Norma. *The Hole in the Dike.*
New York: Crowell, 1975.

Greene, Carol. *The Old Ladies Who
Liked Cats.* New York: Harper Collins, 1991.

Greenfield, Eloise. *Grandpa's Face.*
New York: Putnam, 1988.
—.*Honey, I Love and other Love Poems.*
New York: Harper, 1986.
—.*Nathanial Talking.* New York:
Writers & Readers, 1989.

Hamilton, Virginia. *The People Could
Fly.* New York: Knopf, 1985.

Hartman, Gail. *For Strawberry Jam or
Fireflies.* New York: Bradbury
Press, 1989.

Harvey, Brett. *My Prairie Year.* New
York: Holiday House, 1986.

Havill, Juanita. *Jamaica Tag-Along.*
Boston: Houghton Mifflin, 1989.

Hawkins, Colin. *How Many in This Old
Car?* New York: Putnam, 1988.

Hayes, Sarah. *Clap Your Hands.* New
York: Lothrop, 1988.

Hazen, Barbara Shook. *Tight Times.*
New York: Viking, 1979.

Heide, Florence P. *The Day of Ahmed's
Secret.* New York: Lothrop, 1990.

Hendershot, Judith. *In Coal Country.*
New York: Knopf, 1987.

Henkes, Kevin. *Shhhh.* New York:
Greenwillow, 1989.

Herberman, Ethan. *The City Kids Field Guide*. New York: Simon & Schuster, 1989.

Hill, Eric. *Spot Goes to the Farm*. New York: Putnam, 1987.

—.*Where's Spot*. New York: Putnam, 1990.

Hines, Anna G. *Daddy Makes the Best Spaghetti*. New York: Ticknor & Fields, 1986.

—.*It's Just Me, Emily*. New York: Ticknor & Fields, 1987.

Hirsh, Marilyn. *Could Anything Be Worse?* New York: Holiday House, 1987.

Hoban, Tana. *Of Colors & Things*. New York: Greenwillow, 1989.

Hodges, Margaret. *The Fire Bringer*. Boston: Little, Brown, 1972.

—.*St. George and the Dragon*. Boston: Little, Brown, 1984.

Hort, Lenny. *How Many Stars in the Sky?* New York: Tambourine Books, 1991.

Howard, Katherine. *Little Bunny Follows His Nose*. New York: Western, 1971.

Hughes, Dean. *Making the Team*. New York: Knopf, 1990.

Hughes, Langston. *Don't You Turn Back*. New York: Knopf, 1969.

Hughes, Shirley. *Alfie Gets in First*. New York: Lothrop, 1982.

—.*An Evening at Alfie's*. New York: Lothrop, 1985.

—.*Out and About*. New York: Lothrop, 1988.

Hutchins, Pat. *Rosie's Walk*. New York: Macmillan, 1969.

—.*The Silver Christmas Tree*. New York: Macmillan, 1974.

Inkpen, Mick. *If I Had a Pig*. Boston: Little, Brown, 1988.

Isadora, Rachel. *The Pirates of Bedford Street*. New York: Greenwillow, 1988.

Kalan, Robert. *Jump, Frog, Jump!* New York: Greenwillow, 1981.

Katz, Bobbi. *Poems for Small Friends*. New York: Random House, 1989.

Keats, Ezra Jack. *Peter's Chair*. New York: Harper, 1967.

—.*The Snowy Day*. New York: Viking, 1962.

—.*Whistle for Willie*. New York: Viking, 1964.

Kent, Jack. *There's No Such Thing as a Dragon*. New York: Western, 1975.

Kherdian, David. *Road from Home*. New York: Penguin, 1988.

Kimmel, Eric A. *I Took My Frog To the Library*. New York: Viking, 1990.

Kovalski, Maryann. *The Wheels on the Bus*. Boston: Little, Brown, 1988.

Krasilovsky, Phyllis *The Man Who Did Not Wash His Dishes*. New York: Doubleday, 1950.

Kraus, Robert. *Whose Mouse Are You?* New York: Macmillan, 1972.

Kroll, Steven *The Hokey-Pokey Man*. New York: Holiday House, 1989.

Kunhardt, Dorothy. *Pat The Bunny*. New York: Western, 1942.

Lampton, Christopher. *Stars and Planets*. New York: Doubleday, 1988.

Levinson, Marilyn. *And Don't Bring Jeremy*. New York: Holt, Henry & Co., 1985.

Lewis, Kim. *The Shepherd Boy*. New York: Macmillan, 1990.

Lindbergh, Reeve. *Johnny Appleseed*. Boston: Little, Brown, 1990.

Lionni, Leo. *Swimmy.* New York: Pantheon, 1963.

—.*Tico and the Golden Wings.* New York: Pantheon, 1964.

Lobel, Arnold. *Frog and Toad All Year.* New York: Harper, 1976.

Locker, Thomas. *Family Farm.* New York: Dial, 1988.

—.*Sailing With the Wind.* New York: Dial, 1986.

Lord, Bette Bao. *In the Year of the Boar and Jackie Robinson.* New York: Harper, 1986.

Lowry, Lois. *Anastasia Krupnik.* New York: Bantam, 1984.

—.*Number the Stars.* Boston: Houghton Mifflin, 1989.

—.*A Summer to Die.* Boston: Houghton Mifflin, 1977.

Lyon, David. *The Biggest Truck.* New York: Lothrop, 1988.

Lyon, George Ella. *Come a Tide.* New York: Orchard Books, 1990.

Maass, Robert. *When Autumn Comes.* New York: Holt, Henry & Co., 1990.

MacLachlan, Patricia. *Sarah, Plain and Tall.* New York: Harper, 1985.

Maestro, Betsey. *The Story of the Statue of Liberty.* New York: Morrow, 1989.

Manes, Stephen. *Be a Perfect Person in Just Three Days!* Boston: Houghton Mifflin, 1982.

Manushkin, Fran. *Latkes and Applesauce.* New York: Scholastic, 1990.

Maris, Ron. *Are You There, Bear?* New York: Greenwillow, 1985.

—.*Runaway Rabbit.* New York: Delacorte, 1989.

Martin, Ann M. *Baby Sitters' Club: Kristy's Great Idea.* New York: Scholastic, 1986.

—.*Inside Out.* New York: Scholastic, 1985.

Martin, Bill, Jr. *Brown Bear, Brown Bear, What Do You See?* New York: Holt, Henry & Co., 1983.

Martin, Bill, Jr., and Archambault, John. *Chicka Chicka Boom Boom.* New York: Simon & Schuster, 1989.

—.*Knots on a Counting Rope.* New York: Holt, Henry & Co., 1987.

Marzollo, Jean. *Pretend You're a Cat.* New York: Doubleday, 1990.

McCloskey, Robert. *Blueberries for Sal.* New York: Viking, 1948.

—.*Make Way for Ducklings.* New York: Viking, 1941.

—.*Time of Wonder.* New York: Viking, 1957.

McCue, Lisa *The Little Chick.* New York: Random House, 1986.

McKissack, Patricia. *Flossie and the Fox.* New York: Dial, 1986.

McPhail, David. *Farm Morning.* New York: Harcourt, 1985.

McSwigan, Marie. *Snow Treasure.* New York: Scholastic, 1986.

Modell, Frank. *One Zillion Valentines.* New York: Greenwillow, 1981.

Monrad, Jean. *How Many Kisses Goodnight?* New York: Random House, 1986.

Moore, Elaine. *Grandma's Promise.* New York: Lothrop, 1988.

Mosel, Arlene. *Tikki, Tikki, Tembo.* New York: Holt, 1968.

Myers, Walter D. *The Mouse Rap.* New York: Harper, 1990.

Nichols, Judy. *Storytimes for Two-Year-Olds.* Chicago: ALA, 1987.

O'Dell, Scott. *Island of the Blue Dolphins.* Boston: Houghton Mifflin, 1960.

Ormerod, Jan. *Dad's Back*. New York: Lothrop, 1985.
—.*Just Like Me*. New York: Lothrop, 1986.

Otto, Carolyn. *That Sky, That Rain*. New York: Harper, 1990.

Oxenbury, Helen. *All Fall Down*. New York: Macmillan, 1987.
—.*Clap Hands*.New York: Aladdin, 1987.
—.*Say Goodnight*. New York: Aladdin, 1987.
—.*Tom and Pippo Read a Story*. New York: Macmillan, 1988.

Parish, Peggy. *Amelia Bedelia*. New York: Harper, 1963.
—.*Good Hunting Blue Sky*. New York: Harper, 1989.

Parker, Kristy. *My Dad the Magnificent*. New York: Dutton, 1987.

Peterson, Jeanne. *I Have a Sister, My Sister Is Deaf*. New York: Harper, 1977.

Piper, Watty. *The Little Engine That Could*. New York: Platt & Munk, 1961.

Poems for Fathers. Selected by Myra Cohn Livingston. New York: Holiday House, 1989.

Poems for Mothers. Selected by Myra Cohn Livingston. New York: Holiday House, 1988.

Poems to Read to the Very Young. Selected by Josette Frank. New York: Random House, 1982.

Poetry for Holidays. Selected by Nancy Larrick. Dallas, TX: Garrard, 1966.

Polacco, Patricia. *Thunder Cake*. New York: Putnam, 1990.

Potter, Beatrix. *The Tale of Peter Rabbit*. London: F. Warne & Co., 1903.

Prall, Jo. *My Sister's Special*. Chicago: Childrens, 1985.

Prelutsky, Jack. *Tyrannosaurus Was a Beast*. New York: Greenwillow, 1988.

Radley, Gail. *C.F. In His Corner*. New York: Four Winds Press, 1984.

The Random House Book of Humor for Children. Selected by Pamela Pollock. New York: Random House, 1988.

Rawls, Wilson. *Where the Red Fern Grows*. New York: Doubleday, 1961.

Rey, H.A. *Curious George Rides a Bike*. Boston: Houghton Mifflin, 1952.

Rey, H.A. and Margret Rey. *Curious George Goes to the Hospital*. Boston: Houghton Mifflin, 1966.

Rice, Eve. *Aren't You Coming Too?* New York: Greenwillow, 1988.
—.*Benny Bakes a Cake*. New York: Morrow, 1984.

Richter, Elizabeth. *Losing Someone You Love: When a Brother or Sister Dies*. New York: Putnam, 1986.

Rockwell, Anne. *Bear Child's Book of Special Days*. New York: Dutton, 1989.
—.*My Spring Robin*. New York: Macmillan, 1989.

Rockwell, Anne and Rockwell, Harlow. *Can I Help?* New York: Macmillan, 1982.

Rogers, Paul. *What Will the Weather Be Like Today?* New York: Macmillan, 1990.

Rosen, Michael. *We're Going on a Bear Hunt*. New York: Macmillan, 1989.

Rosenberg, Maxine B. *Finding a Way — Living With Exceptional Brothers and Sisters*. New York: Lothrop, 1988.

Ross, Tony. *Lazy Jack*. New York: Dial, 1986.

Roy, Ron. *Where's Buddy?* Boston: Houghton Mifflin, 1982.

Rylant, Cynthia. *Appalachia: the Voices of Sleeping Birds.* New York: Harcourt, 1991.

—.*Henry and Mudge.* New York: Macmillan, 1990.

—.*The Relatives Came.* New York: Bradbury Press, 1985.

—.*When I Was Young in the Mountains.* New York: Dutton, 1982.

Sanders, Scott Russell. *Aurora Means Dawn.* New York: Bradbury Press, 1989.

Sanford, Doris. *I Can Say No.* Portland, OR: Multnomah Press, 1987.

Say, Allen. *The Lost Lake.* Boston: Houghton Mifflin, 1989.

Schroeder, Alan. *Ragtime Tumpie.* Boston: Little, Brown, 1989.

Schwartz, Amy. *Annabelle Swift, Kindergartner.* New York: Orchard Books, 1988.

Selsam, Millicent. *Keep Looking.* New York: Macmillan, 1989.

Shooter, James C. *After the Dinosaurs.* New York: Western, 1989.

Showers, Paul. *The Listening Walk.* New York: Crowell, 1961.

Shyer, Marlene. *Welcome Home, Jellybean.* New York: Macmillan, 1988.

Siebert, Diane. *Heartland.* New York: Crowell, 1989.
—.*Train Song.* New York: Harper, 1990.

Silverstein, Shel. *Where the Sidewalk Ends.* New York: Harper, 1974.

Slier, Debby. *Me and My Mom.* New York: Checkerboard Press, 1990.

Sobol, Donald J. *Encyclopedia Brown Boy Detective.* New York: Bantam, 1985.

Sobol, Harriet. *My Brother Steven Is Retarded.* New York: Macmillan, 1977.

Soto, Gary. *Baseball in April.* New York: Harcourt, 1990.

Speare, Elizabeth George. *The Sign of the Beaver.* Boston: Houghton Mifflin, 1983.

Sperry, Armstrong. *Call It Courage.* New York: Macmillan, 1940.

Spinelli, Jerry. *Maniac Magee.* Boston: Little, Brown, 1990.

Steele, Mary Q. *Anna's Garden Songs.* New York: Greenwillow, 1989.

Steig, William. *Brave Irene.* New York: Farrar, 1986.

Stolz, Mary. *Storm in the Night.* New York: Harper, 1990.

Surat, Michele Maria. *Angel Child, Dragon Child.* Milwaukee, WI: Raintree, 1983.

Sutherland, Zena. *Orchard Book of Nursery Rhymes.* New York: Orchard Books, 1990.

Svedberg, Ulf. *Nicky, the Nature Detective.* New York: Farrar, 1988.

Taylor, Mark. *Henry Explores the Mountains.* New York: Atheneum, 1975.

Taylor, Mildred D. *Song of the Trees.* New York: Dial, 1975.

Teasdale, Sara. *Collected Poems.* New York: Macmillan, 1966.

Thanksgiving Poems. Selected by Myra Cohn Livingston. New York: Holiday House, 1985.

Thomas, Jane R. *Saying Good-bye to Grandma.* New York: Ticknor & Fields, 1988.

Thompson, Blanche. *All the Silver Pennies.* New York: Macmillan, 1967.

Bibliography 117

Titherington, Jeanne. *Big World, Small World.* New York: Greenwillow, 1985.
—.*Pumpkin, Pumpkin.* New York: Greenwillow, 1986.

Tsutsui, Yoriko. *Anna in Charge.* New York: Viking, 1989.

Turner, Ann. *Street Talk.* Boston: Houghton Mifflin, 1985.

Voight, Cynthia. *Homecoming.* New York: Macmillan, 1981.

Waber, Bernard. *Ira Sleeps Over.* Boston: Houghton Mifflin, 1972.

Watanabe, Shigeo. *How Do I Put It On?* New York: Putnam, 1984.

Wells, Rosemary. *Max's Breakfast.* New York: Dial, 1985.
—.*Noisy Nora.* New York: Dial, 1973.

White, E. B. *Charlotte's Web.* New York: Harper, 1952.

Wildsmith, Brian. *The Owl and the Woodpecker.* New York: Orchard Books, 1971.

Worth, Valerie. *All the Small Poems.* New York: Farrar, 1987.

Yolen, Jane. *Bird Watch.* New York: Philomel Books, 1990.
—.*Owl Moon.* New York: Philomel Books, 1987.

Zion, Gene. *Harry, the Dirty Dog.* New York: Harper, 1956.

Zolotow, Charlotte. *Big Brother.* New York: Harper, 1960.
—.*Do You Know What I'll Do?* New York: Harper, 1958.
—.*If It Weren't For You.* New York: Harper, 1966.
—.*Not a Little Monkey.* New York: Harper, 1989.
—.*Something is Going to Happen.* New York: Harper, 1988.
—.*A Tiger Called Thomas.* New York: Lothrop, 1963.

References

Bernstein, J. and M. Rudman. *Books to Help Children Cope with Separation and Loss: An Annotated Bibliography.* New York: Bowker, 1989.

Cohen, L. "Bibliotherapy: Using Literature to Help Children Deal with Difficult Problems." *Journal of Psychosocial Nursing,* Vol. 25, No. 10, 20-24, 1987.

Cullinan, B. *Literature and the Child.* New York: Harcourt Brace Jovanovich, 1989.

Healy, J. *Endangered Minds: Why Our Children Don't Think.* New York: Simon and Schuster, 1990.

Healy, J. *Your Child's Growing Mind.* New York: Doubleday, 1987.

Hynes A. and M. Hynes-Berry. *Bibliotherapy: The Interactive Process.* Boulder, CO: Westview Press, 1986.

Kobrin, B. *Eyeopeners! How to Choose and Use Children's Books About Real People, Places, and Things.* New York: Viking, 1988.

Koch, K. *Wishes, Lies and Dreams: Teaching Children to Write Poetry.* New York: Chelsea House, 1970.

Matthews, G. "The Institutionalized Child's Need for Library Service." *Library Trends,* Winter, 1978.

Mazza, N. "Poetry and Popular Music as Adjunctive Psychotherapy Techniques." *Innovations in Clinical Practice: A Source Book.* Sarasota, FL: Professional Resource Exchange, 1988.

Mazza et al. "Poetry Therapy with Abused Children." *The Arts in Psychotherapy.* Vol. 14, 85-92, 1987.

McGhee, P. *Humor and Children's Development: A Guide to Practical Applications.* New York: The Haworth Press, 1989.

Morrow, N. 1988. "Poetry By Pediatric Patients." A presentation at the Association for the Care of Children's Health Annual Conference, May, 1988.

Pardeck, J. and J. Pardeck. *Books for Early Childhood: A Developmental Perspective.* Westport, CT: Greenwood, 1988.

Paterson, K. *Gates of Excellence: On Reading and Writing Books for Children.* New York: Dutton, 1988.

Siegel, B. *Love, Medicine and Miracles.* New York: Harper & Row, 1988.

Thompson, C. and L. Rudolph. *Counseling Children.* Belmont, CA: Brooks/Cole Publishing, 1988.

Resources

A. STORY HOUR SUPPORTS

Storytelling and Programming

Bauer, Caroline Feller. *Handbook for Storytellers.* Chicago: ALA, 1977.

de Wit, Dorothy. *Children's Faces Looking Up: Program Building for the Storyteller.* Chicago: ALA, 1979.

Hall, Mary Ann and Pat Hale. *Capture Them with Magic.* Rowayton, CT: New Plays Books, 1982.

Nichols, Judy. *Storytimes for Two-Year-Olds.* Chicago: ALA, 1987.

Painter, William. *Musical Story Hours — Using Music with Storytelling and Puppetry.* Hamden, CT: Library Professional Publications, 1989.

Wilson, Mary. *Representing Children's Book Characters.* Metuchen, NJ: Scarecrow Press, 1989.

Puppetry

Champlin, Connie and Nancy Renfro, *Storytelling with Puppets.* Chicago: ALA, 1985.

Engler, Larry and Carol Fijan. *Making Puppets Come Alive.* New York: Taplinger, 1973.

Latshaw, George. *Puppetry: The Ultimate Disguise.* New York: Richard Rosen Press, 1978.

Renfro, Nancy. *Puppetry and the Art of Story Creation,* Nancy Renfro Studios, 1117 W. 9th St., Austin, TX, 1979.

Cassette Music

Raffi. *Everything Grows*, Troubadour Records, Ltd., 6043 Yonge St., Willowdale, Ontario, Canada, M2M 3W3, 1987.

Raffi and Ken Whiteley. *One Light, One Sun* Troubadour Records, Ltd., 6043 Yonge St., Willowdale, Ontario, Canada M2M 3W3, 1985

Stookey, Paul. *Friends of the Family*, Celebration Shop, Inc., P.O. Box 355, Bedford, TX 76021.

Cutting, Drawing, and Flannel Board Stories

Bauer, Caroline Feller. *Handbook for Storytellers*, pp. 189-202 (flannel board). Chicago: ALA, 1977.

Mallet, Jerry and Marian Bartch. *Stories to Draw*. Hagerstown, MD: Freline Inc., 1982.

Sierra, Judy. *The Flannel Board Storytelling Book*. Bronx, NY: Wilson, 1987.

Stangl, Jean. *Paper Stories: Easy-to-Cut Paper Illustrations that Surprise, Delight, and Captivate*. Belmont, CA: , David S. Lake, 1984.

Finger and Hand Play

Brown, Marc. *Play Rhymes*. New York: Dutton, 1987.

Brown. *Finger Rhymes*. New York: Dutton, 1980.

Brown. *Hand Rhymes*. New York: Dutton, 1985.

Cromwell, Liz. *Finger Frolics*. Livonia, MI: Partner Press, 1976.

Grayson, Marion. *Let's Do Fingerplays*. Bridgeport, CT: Luce, 1962.

Hayes, Sarah. *Clap Your Hands: Finger Rhymes*. New York: Lothrop, Lee and Shepard, 1988.

Sound Filmstrips, Films, and Videos

Weston Woods, Weston, CT 06883. 1-800-243-5020. (All sound filmstrips listed in text are Weston Woods.)

B. SUPPORT READINGS — CHILDREN'S LITERATURE

Binkley, Marilyn. *Becoming a Nation of Readers*. New York: Doubleday, 1987.

Butler, Dorothy. *Babies Need Books*. New York:Atheneum, 1985.

Cullinan, Bernice E. *Literature and the Child — second edition*. San Diego: Harcourt Brace Jovanovich, 1989.

Egoff, Sheila and L. F. Ashley. *Only Connect: Readings in Children's Literature*. New York: Oxford University Press, 1980.

Graves, Ruth. *The RIF Guide to Encouraging Young Readers*. New York: Doubleday, 1987.

Kimmel, Margaret and Elizabeth Segal. *For Reading Out Loud — second edition*. New York: Delacorte, 1988.

Mahoney, Ellen and Leah Wilcox. *Ready, Set, Read: Best Books to Prepare Preschoolers*. Metuchen, NJ: Scarecrow Press, 1985.

Norton, Donna. *Through the Eyes of Children: An Introduction to Children's Literature*. Columbus, OH: Merrill Publishing Co., 1983.

Sutherland, Zena et al. *Children and Books — seventh edition*. Glenview, IL: Scott, Foresman, 1985.

Trelease, Jim. *The Read-Aloud Handbook — third edition*. New York: Penguin, 1989.

C. SUPPORT READINGS — HOSPITALIZED CHILDREN

Anderson, Peggy. *Children's Hospital*. New York: Harper & Row, 1985.

Howe, James. *The Hospital Book*. New York: Crown, 1981.

Krementz, Jill. *How It Feels to Fight for Your Life*. Boston: Little, Brown, 1989.

Plank, Emma. *Working with Children in Hospitals*. Chicago, IL: Year Book Medical Publishers, 1971.

Richter, Elizabeth. *The Teenage Hospital Experience: You Can Handle It*. New York: Coward, McCann, and Geohegan, 1982.

D. BIBLIOTHERAPY — SUGGESTED READINGS

Bernstein, Joanne. *Books to Help Children Cope with Separation and Loss — Vol. 3*. New York: Bowker, 1989.

Brett, Doris. *Annie Stories — A Special Kind of Storytelling*. New York: Workman, 1988.

Cuddigan, Maureen and Mary Beth Hanson. *Growing Pains — Helping Children Deal with Everyday Problems through Reading*. Chicago: ALA, 1988.

Hynes, Arleen and Mary Hynes-Berry. *Bibliotherapy: The Interactive Process*. Boulder: Westview Press, 1986.

E. POETRY WRITING — SUGGESTED READINGS

Journal of Poetry Therapy, Human Sciences Press, 233 Spring St., New York, NY 10013, 1989.

Kennedy, X. J. and Dorothy M. *Knock at a Star: A Child's Introduction to Poetry*. Boston: Little, Brown, 1982.

Koch, Kenneth. *Rose, Where Did You Get that Red?: Teaching Great Poetry to Children*. New York: Random House, 1973.

Koch, Kenneth. *Wishes, Lies and Dreams: Teaching Children to Write Poetry*. New York: Chelsea, 1970.

Kuskin, Karla. *Dogs and Dragons, Trees and Dreams: A Collection of Poems*. New York: Harper & Row, 1980.

Larrick, Nancy. *Let's Do a Poem: Introducing Poetry to Children.* New York: Delacorte, 1991.

McKim, Elizabeth and Judith Steinbergh. *Beyond Words: Writing Poems with Children.* Green Harbor, MA: Wampeter Press, 1983.

Sears, Peter. *Gonna Bake Me a Rainbow Poem.* New York: Scholastic, 1990.

F. ASSOCIATIONS AND ORGANIZATIONS

Association for the Care of Children's Health (ACCH), 7910 Woodmont Ave., Suite 300, Bethesda, MD 20814.

The Children's Literature Center, Library of Congress, 1st St. & Independence Ave. SE, Washington, DC 20540.

The National Association for Poetry Therapy, 225 Williams St., Huron, OH 44839.

National Story League, 555 Tod Ave. NW, Warren, OH 44485 (storytelling).

Puppeteers of America, Inc. Contact through: The Puppetry Store, P.O. Box 3128, Santa Ana, CA 92703.

Reading is Fundamental, Inc. (RIF), P.O. Box 23444, Washington, DC 20026.

Reading Rainbow, GPN, P.O. Box 80669, Lincoln, NE 68501.

Rhea Rubin Consulting, 5860 Heron Dr., Oakland, CA 94618 (415) 339-1274 (bibliotherapy).

G. NEW BOOK SOURCES — DISCOUNTS

Ingram Book Co., 1125 Heil Quaker Blvd., La Vergne, TN 37086, 1-800/937-8000.

Scholastic Inc., Paperbacks for RIF Programs, P.O. Box 7502, 2931 East McCarty St., Jefferson City, MO 65102, 1-800/325-6149.

Story House Corp., Bindery Lane, Charlotteville, NY 12036, 1-800/847-2105.

H. SENSORY IMPAIRED — RESOURCES

Gallaudet Bookstore, Gallaudet University, 800 Florida Ave. NE, Washington, DC 20002, 1-800/422-2546 (hearing impairment).

National Braille Press, 88 Saint Stephen St., Boston, MA 02115, 617/266-6160 (sight impairment).

I. SUPPORT FOR READ-ALOUD VOLUNTEERS

Book Buddies: Volunteers Bring Stories to San Francisco's Hospitalized Children, Children's Services, San Francisco Public Library, Civic Center, San Francisco, CA 94102.

J. PERIODICALS AND JOURNALS — BOOK SELECTION

Booklist, ALA, 50 East Huron St., Chicago, IL 60611.

The Horn Book and *The Horn Book Guide to Children's and Young Adult Books*, 14 Beacon St., Boston, MA 02108, 1-800/325-1170.

Publishers Weekly, Children's Book issues, Magazine Circulation Dept., R. R. Bowker Co., 249 West 17th St., New York, NY 10011.

K. POSTERS, BOOKMARKS, AND OTHER LIBRARY SPECIALTIES

ALA Graphics, 50 East Huron St., Chicago, IL 60611, 1-800/545-2433.

CBC Features, Children's Book Council, P.O. Box 706, 67 Irving Place, New York, NY 10276.

UPSTART, Dept. 18, Box 889, Hagerstown, MD 21741, 1-800/448-4887.

L. GLOSSARY OF MEDICAL TERMS

Bronchopulmonary dysplasia (BPD): a complication of Hyaline Membrane Disease (HMD) related to the use of oxygen and ventilators in treatment.

Comatose: being in a coma; a state of unconsciousness from which the patient cannot be aroused.

Cystic Fibrosis: A genetic disease affecting mucus-secreting cells, particularly those of the lungs. The resulting thickened mucus makes it more difficult for the lungs to stay clear, free of infection, and open for breathing. Cystic fibrosis also damages the glands of the pancreas, which supplies the enzyme needed for fat digestion.

MRI (Magnetic Resonance Imaging): a means of making images of the interior of the body using a strong magnetic field and radio waves rather than x-radiation.

MRI Scan: the process of making an image.

Paraplegia: paralysis of legs and lower part of the body.

Quadriplegia: paralysis of all four limbs.

M. RECOMMENDED BASIC TITLES FOR FAMILY RESOURCE COLLECTION

Bell, Ruth et al. *Changing Bodies, Changing Lives.* New York: Random House, 1988. Teenage sexuality.

Brazelton, T. Berry. *Infants and Mothers,* plus other titles. New York: Dell, 1983. Parenting/growth and development.

Callanan, Charles. *Since Owen.* Baltimore: Johns Hopkins University Press, 1990. Raising a disabled child into adulthood.

Featherstone, Helen. *A Difference in the Family.* New York: Penguin, 1981. Raising a disabled child.

Fraiberg, Selma. *The Magic Years.* New York: Scribner's, 1959. A child's development from birth to age six.

Grollman, Earl A. *Talking About Death: A Dialogue Between Parent and Child.* Boston: Beacon Press, 1990. Picture book format for sharing subject with child plus general text for adults.

Harrison, Helen. *The Premature Baby Book.* New York: St. Martin's Press, 1983. A parent's guide.

Hausher, Rosemarie. *Children and the AIDS Virus: A Book for Children, Parents, and Teachers.* New York: Clarion, 1989. Explanation of the body's immune system, the AIDS virus attack on the system, and methods of prevention.

Jones, Monica. *Home Care for the Chronically Ill or Disabled Child.* New York: Harper & Row, 1985. A parent's guide.

Krementz, Jill. *How It Feels to Fight for Your Life.* New York: Little, Brown, 1989. Interviews with photographs of children and adolescents with disabilities, traumas, and chronic illnesses.

McCollum, Audrey T. *The Chronically Ill Child: A Guide for Parents and Professionals.* New York: Yale University Press, 1981. A helpful reference resource.

Mellonie, Bryand and Robert Ingpen. *Lifetimes.* New York: Bantam, 1983. Explanation of death presented in beautiful picture book format.

Silverstein, Herma. *Teen Guide to Single Parenting.* New York: Franklin Watts, 1989. A readable guide for the young parent on child raising from birth to two years.

Simons, Robin. *After the Tears.* San Diego: Harcourt Brace Jovanovich, 1987. Raising a disabled child.

Author/Title Index

Subject Index

American Library Association (ALA), 17, 65

Association for the Care of Children's Health (ACCH), 81-82, 88, 99

Bibliotherapy

    approaches, 67, 68
    case studies, 53-59, 67-68, 69-71
    definition, 65
    usage, 67, 91

Book cart

    coping skills with ill patients, 63-64
    environment on patient divisions, 61, 64
    services,   61, 63, 92

Book Collection

    interlibrary loan from public library, 1, 7, 101
    new books, 7, 87
    start-up purchases, 7
    title selection, 7-16, 92
    used books, 1, 4

Book plate, 5

Child life specialist, work with patients, 4, 47, 65, 91

Children with special needs

    bibliotherapy/reading aloud, 69-71
    chronically ill, xv, 47
    comatose, 56-57
    developmentally delayed, 56
    dying, 58
    head injured, 55

    hearing impaired, 53
    neurologically devastated, 57-58
    quadriplegic, 54-55
    terminally ill, 58
    ventilator dependent, 59-60
    vision impaired, 54

Collection, organization of books

    cataloging, 4
    circulation, 5
    losses, 5
    return, 5
    shelving, 4, 7

Comatose, see Children with special needs

Community outreach, 4, 85-88

Developmentally delayed, see Children with special needs

Family resource collection

    circulation, 83
    definition, 81
    guidelines, 81-83
    promotion, 101
    users, 83, 92

Funding, sources of

    continuing, 2
    start-up, 2

Glossary of medical terms, 126

Grandparents, 93-95

Hannigan, Margaret, 65